MW01014957

LAND BETWEEN THE LAKES

OUTDOOR HANDBOOK

Your Complete Guide for Hiking, Camping, Fishing,
and Nature Study in Western Tennessee and Kentucky

PLYMOUTH PUBLIC LIBRARY
PLYMOUTH IN 46563

OTHER BOOKS BY JOHNNY MOLLOY

50 Hikes in Alabama

50 Hikes in the Ozarks

50 Hikes in the North Georgia Mountains

50 Hikes in South Carolina

50 Hikes on Tennessee's Cumberland Plateau

60 Hikes Within 60 Miles: San Antonio &
Austin (with Tom Taylor)

60 Hikes Within 60 Miles: Nashville

A Canoeing & Kayaking Guide to the Streams
of Kentucky (with Bob Sehlinger)

A Paddler's Guide to Everglades National Park

Backcountry Fishing: A Guide for Hikers,
Backpackers and Paddlers

Beach & Coastal Camping in Florida

Beach & Coastal Camping in the Southeast

Best Easy Day Hikes: Chapel Hill

Best Easy Day Hikes: Charleston, South Carolina

Best Easy Day Hikes: Cincinnati

Best East Day Hikes: Greensboro/
Winston-Salem

Best Easy Day Hikes: Jacksonville

Best Easy Day Hikes: Madison, Wisconsin

Best Easy Day Hikes: New River Gorge

Best Easy Day Hikes: Richmond

Best Easy Day Hikes: Tallahassee

Best Easy Day Hikes: Tampa Bay

Best Hikes Near Cincinnati

Best Hikes Near Columbus

Best Hikes Near Raleigh, Durham &
Chapel Hill

Best Hikes of the Appalachian Trail: South

Best Tent Camping: The Carolinas

Best Tent Camping: Colorado

Best Tent Camping: Georgia

Best Tent Camping: Kentucky

Best Tent Camping: Southern Appalachian &
Smoky Mountains

Best Tent Camping: Tennessee

Best Tent Camping: West Virginia

Best Tent Camping: Wisconsin

Can't Miss Hikes in North Carolina's
National Forests

Day & Overnight Hikes on Kentucky's
Sheltowee Trace

Day & Overnight Hikes in West Virginia's
Monongahela National Forest

Day Hiking Southwest Florida

Five-Star Trails: Chattanooga

Five-Star Trails: Knoxville

Five-Star Trails: Roanoke

Five-Star Trails: Tri-Cities of Tennessee
and Virginia

From the Swamp to the Keys: A Paddle through
Florida History

Hiking the Florida Trail: 1,100 Miles, 78 Days
and Two Pairs of Boots

Hiking Mississippi

Hiking Through History: New England

Hiking Through History: Virginia

Mount Rogers National Recreation Area
Guidebook

The Hiking Trails of Florida's National Forests,
Parks, and Preserves

Long Trails of the Southeast

Outward Bound Canoeing Handbook

Paddling Georgia

Paddling South Carolina

Paddling Tennessee

Top Trails: Great Smoky Mountains
National Park

Top Trails: Shenandoah National Park

Trial By Trail: Backpacking in the Smoky
Mountains

Waterfall Hiking Tennessee

Waterfalls of the Blue Ridge

LAND BETWEEN
THE LAKES

OUTDOOR HANDBOOK

Your Complete Guide for Hiking, Camping, Fishing,
and Nature Study in Western Tennessee and Kentucky

JOHNNY MOLLOY
2ND EDITION

PLYMOUTH PUBLIC LIBRARY
PLYMOUTH IN 46563

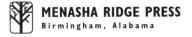
MENASHA RIDGE PRESS
Birmingham, Alabama

LAND BETWEEN THE LAKES OUTDOOR HANDBOOK: YOUR COMPLETE GUIDE FOR HIKING, CAMPING, FISHING, AND NATURE STUDY IN WESTERN TENNESSEE AND KENTUCKY

Copyright © 2016 by Johnny Molloy
All rights reserved
Printed in the United States of America
Published by Menasha Ridge Press
Distributed by Publishers Group West
Second edition, first printing

Library of Congress Cataloging-in-Publication Data
Names: Molloy, Johnny, 1961-
Title: Land Between the Lakes outdoor handbook : your complete guide for
    hiking, camping, fishing, horseback riding, nature study and more / Johnny
    Molloy.
Other titles: Land Between the Lakes National Recreation Area handbook
Description: Second Edition. | Birmingham, Alabama : Menasha Ridge Press,
    [2016] | "Distributed by Publishers Group West"—T.p. verso. | Includes
    index.
Identifiers: LCCN 2015051019| ISBN 9781634040648 | ISBN 9781634040655 (Ebook)
Subjects: LCSH: Outdoor recreation—Land Between the Lakes (Ky. and
    Tenn.)—Guidebooks. | Land Between the Lakes (Ky. and Tenn.)—Guidebooks.
Classification: LCC GV191.42.L36 M65 2016 | DDC 796.50976—dc23
LC record available at http://lccn.loc.gov/2015051019

Cover design: Scott McGrew
Text design: Annie Long
Maps: Steve Jones and Johnny Molloy
Cover and interior photos by Johnny Molloy unless otherwise noted
Indexing: Rich Carlson

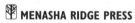 **MENASHA RIDGE PRESS**
An imprint of AdventureKEEN
2204 First Ave. S, Ste. 102
Birmingham, AL 35233

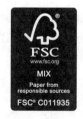
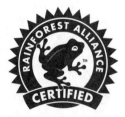

Visit **menasharidge.com** for a complete listing of our books and for ordering information. Contact us at our website, at **facebook.com/menasharidge**, at **twitter.com/menasharidge**, or at **blog.menasharidge .com** with questions or comments.

▪ Contents ▪

■ Part Four: SEEING THE REST OF THE PARK   146

■ LIST OF MAPS

Legend

○ Canton	KENTUCKY	80	68	520 100	
City	State border	Interstate	US hwy	Other roads	Trails

- Boat ramp
- Campsite
- Cemetery
- Dam
- Drinking water
- Heritage interpretive marker
- HM Heritage marker
- Hiking trailhead
- P Parking
- Park office

- Phone access
- Picnic area
- Point of interest
- Restroom
- Scenic view
- Shelter
- Shooting range
- Stone furnace
- Trash/dumpster
- Water access

• Acknowledgments •

THANKS TO MY WIFE, KERI ANNE, for her help at home and on the trail. Thanks to Kelty for providing tents, sleeping bags, and more essential outdoor equipment, and thanks to Oboz for providing fine hiking shoes on the trail. Thanks to all the staffers past and present at Land Between The Lakes National Recreation Area, from those who developed the park when it was part of TVA and forward to today's employees who make this slice of the South a scenic destination for us to enjoy.

Entrance sign along Woodlands Trace

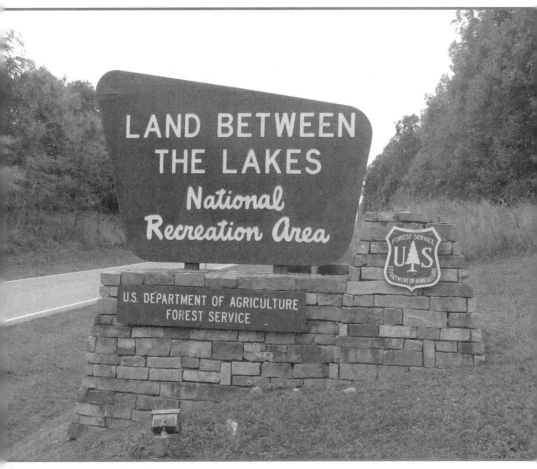

Land Between The Lakes
National Recreation Area

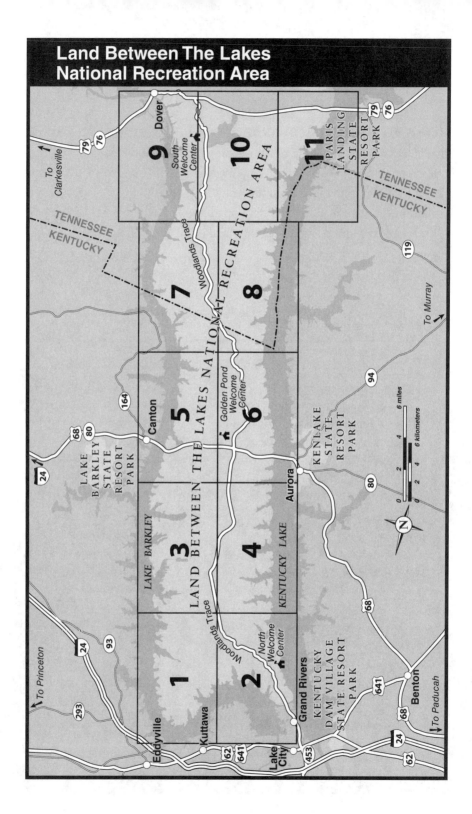

Map 1

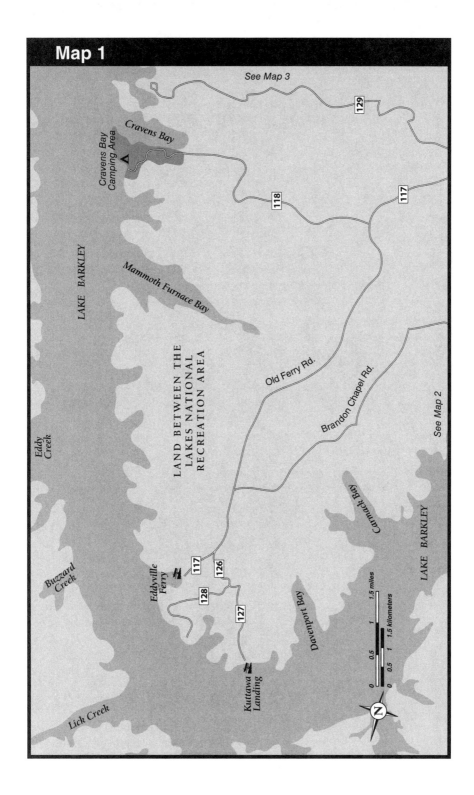

See Map 3

129

Cravens Bay

Cravens Bay Camping Area

118

117

LAKE BARKLEY

Mammoth Furnace Bay

LAND BETWEEN THE LAKES NATIONAL RECREATION AREA

Old Ferry Rd.

Brandon Chapel Rd.

See Map 2

Eddy Creek

Buzzard Creek

Eddyville Ferry

117

126

128

127

Carnuck Bay

LAKE BARKLEY

Davenport Bay

Kuttawa Landing

Lick Creek

0   0.5   1   1.5 miles

0   0.5   1   1.5 kilometers

N

Map 2

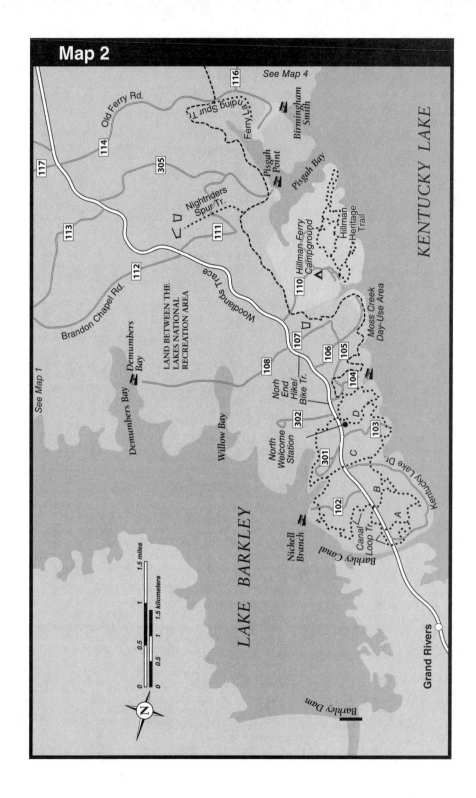

See Map 4

KENTUCKY LAKE

Old Ferry Rd.

Ferry Ln.

Landing Spur Tr.

116

Birmingham Smith

Pisgah Point

Pisgah Bay

114

305

117

Nightriders Spur Tr.

Hillman Heritage Trail

113

111

Hillman-Ferry Campground

112

110

Brandon Chapel Rd.

Moss Creek Day-Use Area

Woodlands Trace

107

Demumbers Bay

LAND BETWEEN THE LAKES NATIONAL RECREATION AREA

108

106

105

See Map 1

North End Hike/Bike Tr.

104

302

D

Willow Bay

North Welcome Station

103

301

C

B

Kentucky Lake Dr.

102

A

Nickell Branch

Canal Loop Tr.

Barkley Canal

LAKE BARKLEY

1.5 miles

1.5 kilometers

0.5   1

0.5   1

0   0

N

Barkley Dam

Grand Rivers

xiv

Map 3

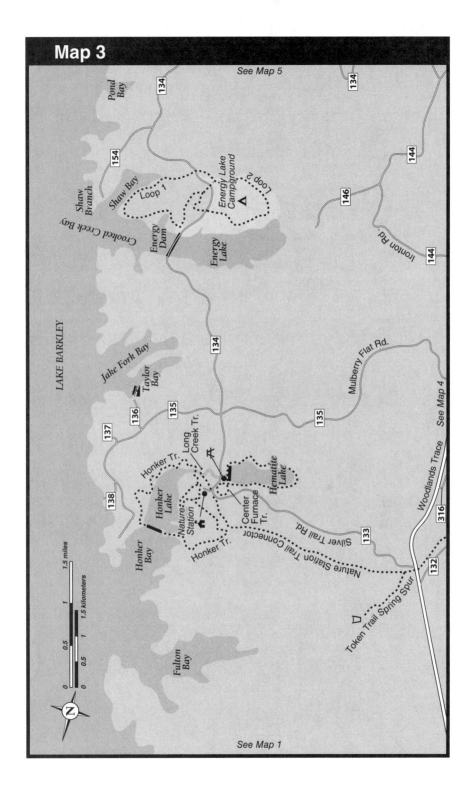

Map 4

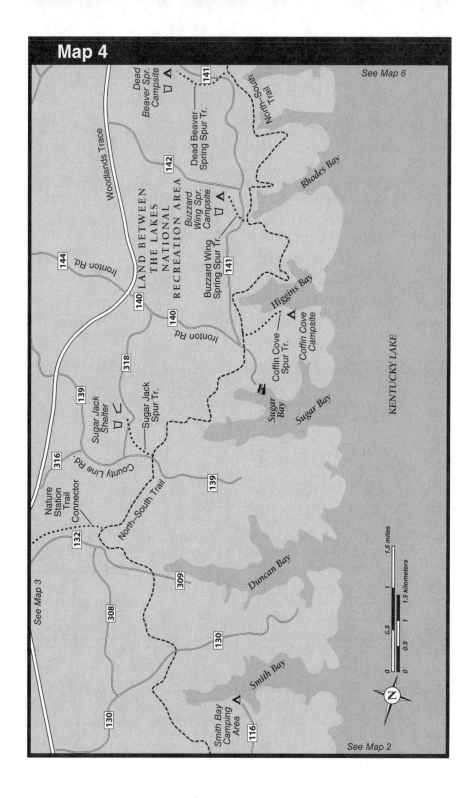

See Map 6
See Map 3
See Map 2

Dead Beaver Spr. Campsite

Dead Beaver Spring Spur Tr.

North-South Trail

Rhodes Bay

Woodlands Trace

LAND BETWEEN THE LAKES NATIONAL RECREATION AREA

142

Buzzard Wing Spr. Campsite

Ironton Rd.

144

Buzzard Wing Spring Spur Tr.

141

Higgins Bay

140

140

Ironton Rd.

Coffin Cove Spur Tr.

Coffin Cove Campsite

KENTUCKY LAKE

318

Sugar Jack Shelter

Sugar Jack Spur Tr.

139

Sugar Bay

Sugar Bay

316

County Line Rd.

139

Nature Station Trail Connector

North-South Trail

Duncan Bay

132

309

308

130

Smith Bay

130

Smith Bay Camping Area

116

0.5   1   1.5 miles

0   0.5   1   1.5 kilometers

N

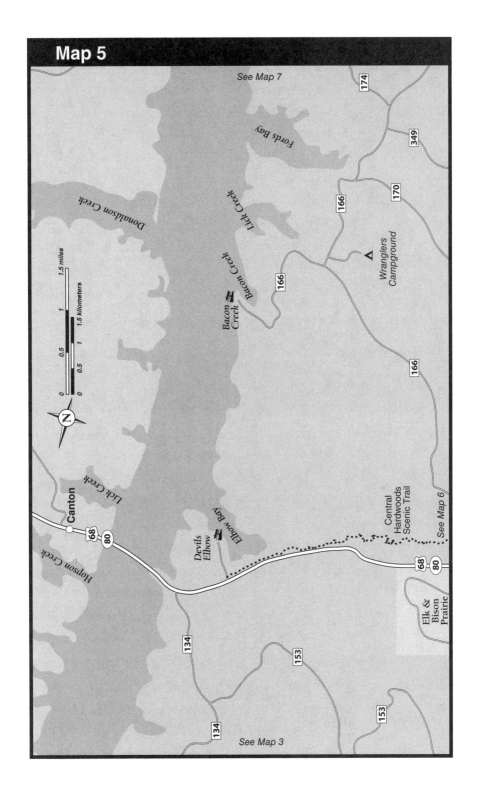

Map 5

See Map 7

174

349

166

170

Wranglers Campground

166

166

Fords Bay

Lick Creek

Bacon Creek

Bacon Creek

Donaldson Creek

1.5 miles
0.5   1
0   1   1.5 kilometers
0.5   1
0   1

N

Canton

Lick Creek

Hopson Creek

68
80

Devils Elbow

Elbow Bay

Central Hardwoods Scenic Trail

See Map 6

68
80

Elk & Bison Prairie

134

153

134

153

See Map 3

Map 6

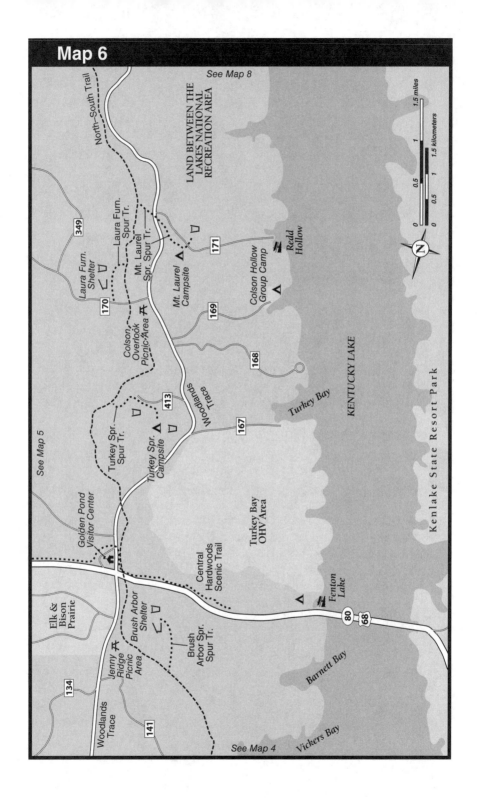

See Map 8

LAND BETWEEN THE LAKES NATIONAL RECREATION AREA

North–South Trail

349

Laura Furn. Shelter

Laura Furn. Spur Tr.

Mt. Laurel Spr. Spur Tr.

170

Colson Overlook Picnic Area

171

Redd Hollow

Colson Hollow Group Camp

Mt. Laurel Campsite

169

168

KENTUCKY LAKE

See Map 5

413

Turkey Spr. Spur Tr.

Woodlands Trace

167

Turkey Bay

Turkey Spr. Campsite

Golden Pond Visitor Center

Turkey Bay OHV Area

Kenlake State Resort Park

Elk & Bison Prairie

Jenny Ridge Picnic Area

Brush Arbor Shelter

Central Hardwoods Scenic Trail

Fenton Lake

80

68

134

Brush Arbor Spr. Tr.

Woodlands Trace

141

Barnett Bay

See Map 4

Vickers Bay

1.5 miles

1.5 kilometers

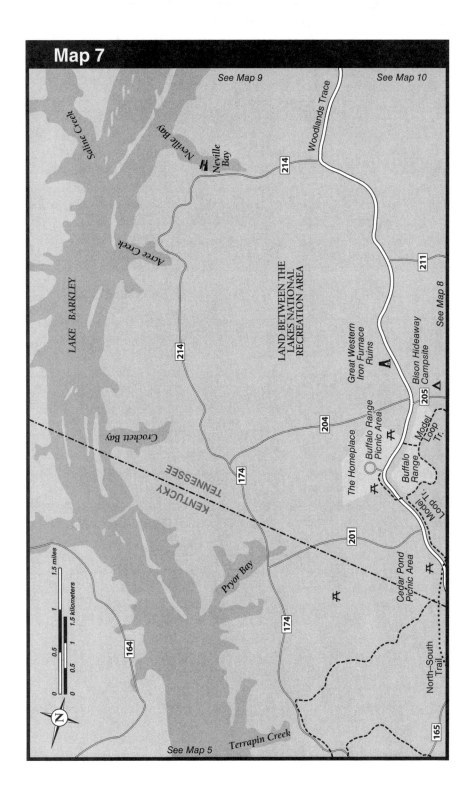

Map 7

See Map 9

See Map 10

Woodlands Trace

Saline Creek

Neville Bay

Neville Bay

214

Acree Creek

LAKE BARKLEY

LAND BETWEEN THE
LAKES NATIONAL
RECREATION AREA

214

211

See Map 8

Great Western
Iron Furnace
Ruins

Bison Hideaway
Campsite

205

Crockett Bay

204

Buffalo Range
Picnic Area

The Homeplace

Model
Loop
Tr.

KENTUCKY
TENNESSEE

174

Buffalo
Range

Model
Loop Tr.

201

Pryor Bay

Cedar Pond
Picnic Area

1.5 miles

1.5 kilometers

1

0.5

1

0

0.5

0

174

164

North–South
Trail

165

N

See Map 5

Terrapin Creek

Map 8

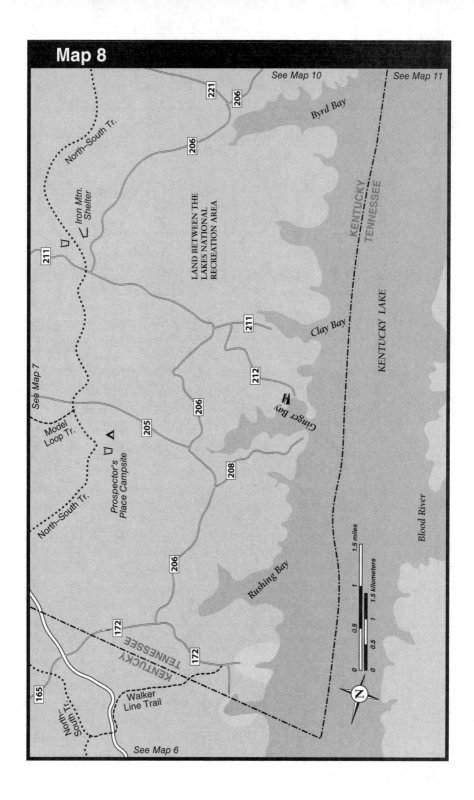

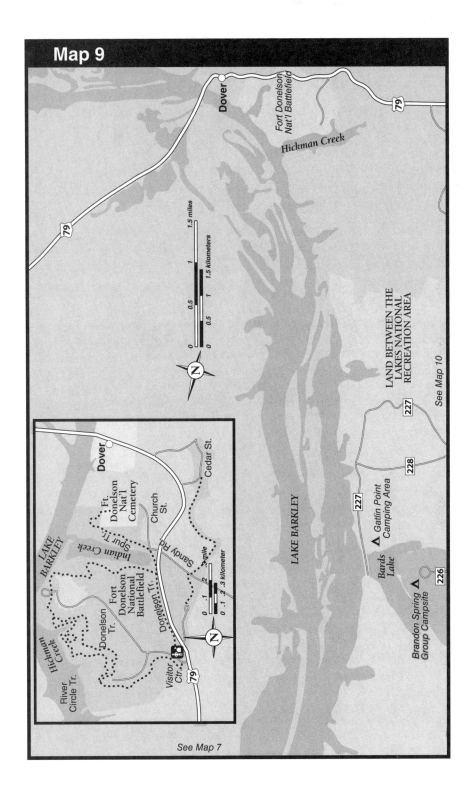

Map 9

Dover

Fort Donelson
Nat'l Battlefield

79

Hickman Creek

1.5 miles
1
0.5
0
1.5 kilometers
1
0.5
0

N

LAND BETWEEN THE
LAKES NATIONAL
RECREATION AREA

See Map 10

227

228

227

▲ Gatlin Point
Camping Area

LAKE BARKLEY

Bards
Lake

Brandon Spring ▲
Group Campsite

226

Dover

Ft.
Donelson
Nat'l
Cemetery

Church
St.

Cedar St.

LAKE
BARKLEY

Indian Creek
Spur Tr.

Sandy Rd.

.3mile

Donelson Tr.

Fort
Donelson
National
Battlefield

Donelson
Tr.

.3 kilometer
.2
.1
0
.2
.1
0

Hickman
Creek

N

River
Circle Tr.

Visitor
Ctr.

79

See Map 7

xxi

Map 10

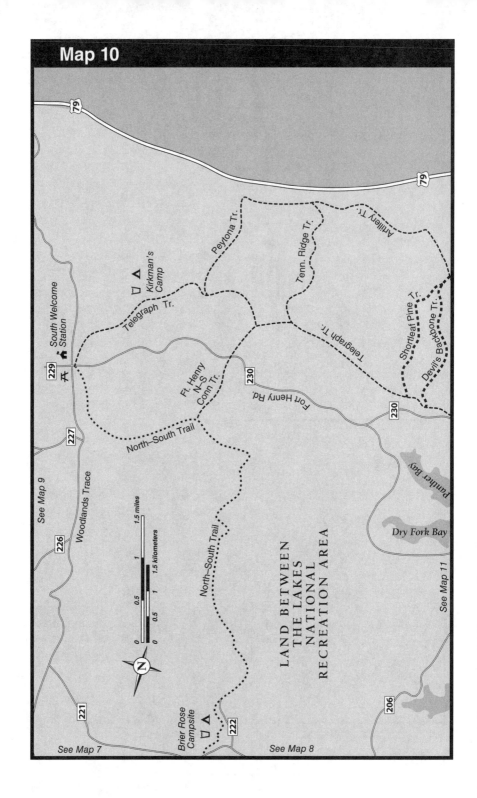

LAND BETWEEN
THE LAKES
NATIONAL
RECREATION AREA

Kirkman's Camp

South Welcome Station

Telegraph Tr.

Peytona Tr.

Tenn. Ridge Tr.

Artillery Tr.

Telegraph Tr.

Shortleaf Pine Tr.

Devil's Backbone Tr.

Ft. Henry N-S Conn Tr.

Fort Henry Rd

North-South Trail

Woodlands Trace

North-South Trail

North-South Trail

Panther Bay

Dry Fork Bay

Brier Rose Campsite

See Map 9

See Map 7

See Map 8

See Map 11

79

229

227

226

221

230

230

222

206

1.5 miles

1.5 kilometers

0.5   1

0.5   1

0   0

N

Map 11

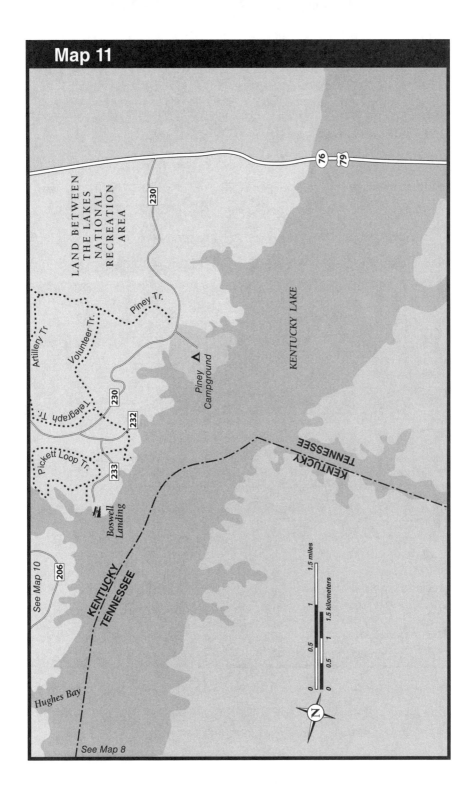

Map 12: Hillman Heritage Trail

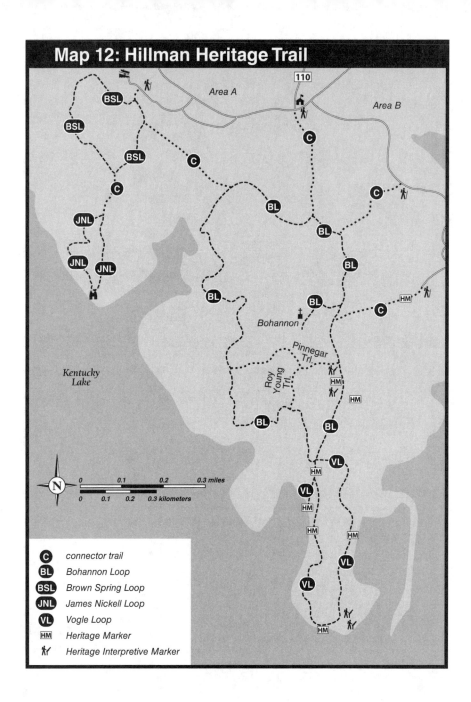

Area A

Area B

110

BSL

BSL

BSL

C

C

C

C

JNL

BL

BL

JNL JNL

BL

BL

BL

HM

C

Bohannon

Pinnegar Trl.

Kentucky Lake

Roy Young Trl.

HM

HM

HM

BL

BL

BL

VL

HM

VL

HM

HM

HM

VL

VL

HM

C connector trail
BL Bohannon Loop
BSL Brown Spring Loop
JNL James Nickell Loop
VL Vogle Loop
HM Heritage Marker
Ŕ Heritage Interpretive Marker

N

0   0.1   0.2   0.3 miles

0   0.1   0.2   0.3 kilometers

Map 13: Central Hardwoods Scenic Trail

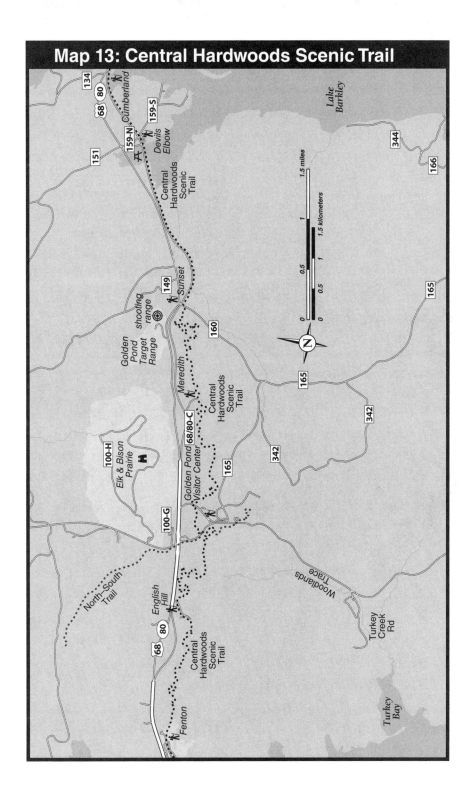

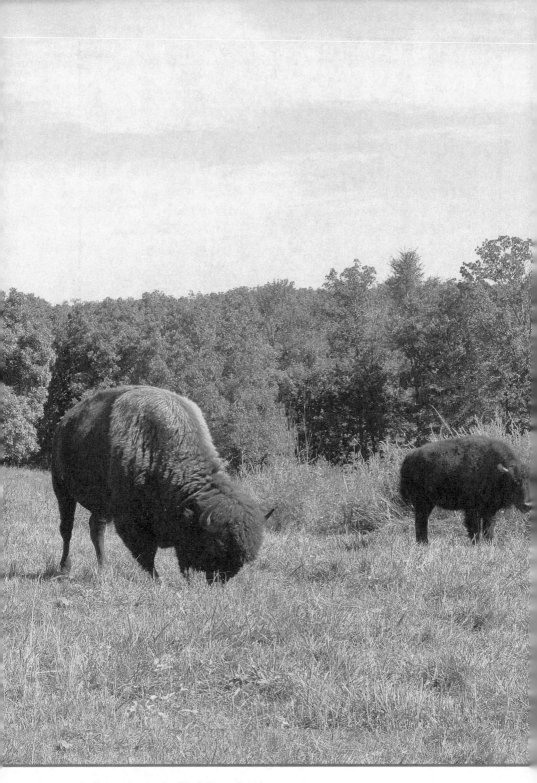

Buffalo graze at the Elk & Bison Prairie.

· Introduction ·

History of LBL

LAND BETWEEN THE Lakes National Recreation Area is a treasure not only to the states of Tennessee and Kentucky, but also to the Mid-American region. Look at a map: LBL covers more than 170,000 contiguous acres of protected lands nestled on a peninsula between the Tennessee and Cumberland Rivers. To find a swath of protected land that size you have to look east all the way to the Great Smoky Mountains National Park or west to the massive national forests of the Rocky Mountains. The only other nearby federal lands that compare in size are Illinois's Shawnee National Forest or Arkansas's Ouachita National Forest. A closer look, though, at these impressive, neighboring lands reveals an agglomeration of individual tracts, not a contiguous piece such as exists at Land Between The Lakes.

This peninsula, running north–south between the Tennessee and Cumberland Rivers, was once the home of the Shawnee Indians, who hunted buffalo and other animals in the hardwood hollows and hickory-oak ridges. The first white pioneers came here to settle land grants earned during the Revolutionary War. They found the creek bottoms rich for planting and the rivers easy for transporting their excess agricultural products. They dubbed the region Between The Rivers. These rivers were at the same time impediments, as bridges crossing them were centuries away in coming. But settlers came anyway, and the Shawnee were soon gone, a result of the Indian Removal Act of 1830.

The rush westward continued and Between The Rivers became a backwater, developing its own culture, yet stayed connected to the outside by the rivers that formed its borders. Iron ore was found in quantity, and great iron furnaces sprang up in the region, using the vast timber, water, and limestone resources to transform the ore into production iron. Practical products such as kettles, nails, and other useful items were forged and sold in the region, but most iron was sent up north via the rivers.

Many Between The Rivers residents weren't sure if they were in Kentucky or Tennessee when the Civil War broke out, an important bit of information since Kentucky chose neutrality and Tennessee sided with the Confederacy.

1

The Union saw the Tennessee and Cumberland Rivers as watery gateways to invade the South. They aimed to use the rivers as supply and troop routes and as a wedge to split the Confederacy in half. The battles at Fort Henry, on the Tennessee River, and Fort Donelson, on the Cumberland River, brought fighting to the region and mayhem for the rest of the war, as Federal soldiers and guerrillas with allegiances to no one raided homes and towns in search of food and supplies.

The war ended and the iron production died with it. Between The Rivers spent the last half of the nineteenth century recovering from the Civil War. Once again, the area slipped to the rear of the American stage. Then the Tennessee Valley Authority (TVA) came to be. Authorized during the Great Depression of the 1930s, this federal entity set about building dams for flood control and "developing" the Tennessee River Valley. Kentucky Dam was built between 1938 and 1944, backing up the Tennessee River and flooding the lands on the west side of Between The Rivers. Family homes and farms were bought out and the people removed before the gates were closed. Later, TVA built more dams. One dam in particular, Barkley Dam on the Cumberland River, would still the waters on the east side of Between The Rivers. Somebody at TVA saw the swath of land between a dammed Cumberland and Tennessee as a vast recreation area, despite many folks living there. Momentum built, and the TVA, buoyed by John F. Kennedy's 1961 speech emphasizing the need for acquiring federal lands for recreation, sprang into action.

Then, in a story similar to the creation of the Great Smoky Mountains National Park, citizens of the Between The Rivers area were forced to sell their lands. Some were happy to go, most weren't, and still others felt they didn't receive fair market value for their land. However, by 1969, TVA was running Land Between The Lakes as a recreation demonstration project.

Meanwhile, Lake Barkley was filled and a canal was built connecting Lake Barkley and Kentucky Lake. Then Land Between The Lakes was protected in a watery swaddle on three sides. In addition, these lakes enhanced recreation opportunities at Land Between The Lakes. Irregular budgets made managing Land Between The Lakes a challenge for TVA. In 1999, Congress decided that the U.S. Forest Service and the Department of Agriculture should manage Land Between the Lakes. Today, the Forest Service is doing a fine job in managing this land using the multiple-use concept. Visitors are growing in their appreciation of Land Between The Lakes, and most residents, once embittered over having their land taken from them, are now seeing Land Between The Lakes as a source of pride as sightseers from all over the United States visit a place we can all hold dear.

Recreation Overview

LAND BETWEEN THE Lakes National Recreation Area (LBL) truly lives up to its name. Recreation opportunities abound: camping, fishing, hiking, nature study, horseback riding, swimming, mountain biking, historical study, pleasure boating, scenic driving, wildlife observation, paddling, road biking, and off-roading.

Spread over a 40-mile-long peninsula, varying between 1 and 9 miles wide, the size of LBL is an impressive 171,280 acres. Additionally, the vast lake acreage on either side of the land broadens opportunities here. But this area is more than just land and lakes. Several unique features broaden LBL's appeal. In the south, there is The Homeplace, a living history farm where interpreters dressed in period clothing live as area residents did back in the 1850s. The South Bison Range is nearby. Here one of two herds of buffalo live and reproduce as they did centuries ago. The Golden Pond Planetarium at the main visitor center offers a glimpse into the night sky, explaining the heavens above. The Elk & Bison Prairie is a restored "barren" where elk and bison live in an ecosystem like that in western Kentucky before the United States was even a country. The Nature Station is an environmental education area where visitors interact with the animals of LBL. Here, staff explain how the land and animals form the web of life and lead guided events exploring different threads in this web, including eagle-watching tours.

Camping is a premium land activity in LBL. The land sports a whopping 1,427 campsites. Nine developed campgrounds complement the nearly limitless backcountry camping opportunities. Campers can enjoy hot showers or rough it. Or they camp with like-minded folks, as the equestrians do at Wranglers Camp. The horseback riders also enjoy their own trail system, with 106 miles of bridle paths.

Other trail enthusiasts will find pathways for them. Hikers and mountain bikers can enjoy the North–South Trail, the master path of the LBL trail system. This trail runs over 60 miles along the peninsula between the lakes. Many paths spur off the North–South Trail. Other trail systems lie within the recreation area confines. The Fort Henry Trails run through the hills and hollows of the south end, allowing hikers to retrace the footsteps of Civil War soldiers who fought here, as do the nearby Fort Donelson National Battlefield Trails. The Nature Station Trails are rounded out with environmental education opportunities along the paths. The Canal Loop Trails are developed for mountain bikers, and road bikers pedal the many paved roads of LBL.

And there are the lakes. The canal linking Kentucky Lake and Lake Barkley together makes them one of the largest man-made bodies of water in the world. It is on these lakes where anglers vie for crappie, bass, bluegill, and catfish. Fishing is big here. LBL has 26 boat ramps, which make getting on the water easy. Others enjoy the water simply to boat, swim, or relax in the cool water on a hot day. A few others will be paddling by canoe or sea kayak, looking out on the 300 miles of natural, undeveloped shoreline that LBL offers. Other smaller lakes and ponds lie within the confines of LBL, adding more scenic fishing, swimming, and paddling opportunities.

Yet there is more: visitors can picnic, they can backpack, and they can camp together in group facilities. This book will spare you the tiring and sometimes frustrating effort of researching all of the opportunities to be found at Land Between The Lakes National Recreation Area and leave you time to enjoy all of the beauty this swath of Tennessee and Kentucky has to offer.

Land Between The Lakes Weather

THE CLIMATE AT Land Between The Lakes is seasonal, with warm to hot summers and moderate winters. Early spring is the most variable, with periodic warm-ups, broken by cold fronts bringing rain then chilly temperatures. Later, temperatures stay warm and become hot by July. Typically, mornings start clear, then clouds build and hit-or-miss thunderstorms occur by afternoon. The first cool fronts hit LBL around mid-September. Fall sees warm, clear days and cool nights with the least amount of rain, though rain amounts are somewhat steady throughout the year. Precipitation picks up in November, and temperatures generally stay cool to cold, broken by occasional mild spells. Snowfall varies from winter to winter but averages less than 15 inches per year.

WEATHER AVERAGES

	AVERAGE HIGH	AVERAGE LOW	MEAN TEMPERATURE	AVERAGE PRECIPITATION
JANUARY	41°F	22°F	32°F	3.8"
FEBRUARY	47°F	25°F	36°F	4.3"
MARCH	58°F	35°F	47°F	5.3"
APRIL	69°F	44°F	57°F	4.7"
MAY	77°F	53°F	66°F	4.8"
JUNE	86°F	61°F	74°F	3.5"
JULY	86°F	65°F	78°F	4.4"
AUGUST	88°F	64°F	76°F	3.4"
SEPTEMBER	82°F	57°F	70°F	3.5"
OCTOBER	71°F	44°F	58°F	3.2"
NOVEMBER	58°F	36°F	48°F	4.9"
DECEMBER	46°F	26°F	37°F	5.1"

About This Guidebook

THIS BOOK COMPREHENSIVELY and systematically covers nearly every potential outdoor activity at Land Between The Lakes National Recreation Area. For starters, every visitor facility is thoroughly covered. The visitor facilities offer unique opportunities at LBL, such as visiting the historic Homeplace, the Nature Station, or the Golden Pond Planetarium. For hikers, every marked and maintained trail is detailed. Beyond the trails are various other activities at LBL, such as fishing, swimming, scenic driving, picnicking, camping, and touring. The "Swim Beaches" section includes an overview of the swimming area, what it is like, and directions for accessing the beach.

The "Scenic Drives" section details some great auto touring trips of the recreation area. There are not only paved auto tours but also forest drives that traverse some of the lesser-used gravel roads of LBL. Each description includes the type of road, the length of the auto tour, highlights to be seen along the tour, and amenities to be found along the tour. Picnic areas are also described with an overview of what the picnic area is like, along with how to get to the picnic area and nearby activities.

The "Places to Lay Your Head" section details campgrounds and area resorts. Recreation area campgrounds are reviewed using at-a-glance information that includes when open, number of campsites, site amenities, site assignment, facilities, and fees. A narrative follows, describing the campground setting and area activities, along with access directions. Horseback riding is popular at LBL, and there is a special camp for equestrians. The same goes for off-road driving enthusiasts. These are also included in the campground section. Nearby state parks are detailed not only for camping facilities but also for most developed lodging and indoor and outdoor activities.

Hopefully, this book will lead you to appreciate and enjoy the Land Between The Lakes National Recreation Area so much that you will want to volunteer to keep it a great place. In case this happens, contact information is included in the appendix.

LAND BETWEEN THE LAKES TRAIL TABLE						
	TYPE	DIFFICULTY	LENGTH	USE	MAP	PAGE
CANAL LOOP TRAILS						
Canal Loop Trail	F, B	M to D	10.8	H	2	59
North Paved Trail	F, B	E	1.5	H	2	63
Trail Connector A	F, B	E	0.5	M to H	2	64
Trail Connector B	F, B	E	0.5	M	2	64
Trail Connector C	F, B	E	0.7	M to H	2	65
Trail Connector D	F, B	E	0.8	H	2	66
HILLMAN HERITAGE TRAIL						
Bohannon Loop	F, B	M	2.1	H	12	68
Vogle Loop	F, B	M	1.0	M	12	68
Brown Spring Loop	F, B	M	0.7	H	12	69
James Nickell Loop	F, B	M	0.5	H	12	69
CENTRAL HARDWOODS SCENIC TRAIL						
CHST: Fenton to Cumberland	F, B	M	11	H	13	70
ENERGY LAKE TRAILS						
Loop 1	F only	M	3.9	L	3	74
Loop 2	F only	M	2.1	M	3	75
FORT DONELSON NATIONAL BATTLEFIELD TRAILS						
Donelson Trail	F only	M	3.1	M	9	77
Earthworks Trail	F only	E to M	1.3	L	9	79

LAND BETWEEN THE LAKES TRAIL TABLE

	TYPE	DIFFICULTY	LENGTH	USE	MAP	PAGE
River Circle Trail	F only	E to M	1.1	L to M	9	81
Spur Trail	F only	E	1.3	L	9	82
FORT HENRY AREA TRAILS						
Artillery Trail	F only	M	3.2	L to M	11	83
Boswell Trail	F only	E	0.4	M	11	84
Devils Backbone Trail	F only	M	1.5	M	11	85
Peytona Trail	F only	M	3.0	M	11	86
Picket Loop Trail	F only	M	3.6	M	11	87
Piney Trail	F only	M	2.3	M	11	89
Telegraph Trail	F only	M to D	7.5	M	11	90
Telegraph-Pickett Trail	F only	E	0.3	M	11	93
Tennessee Ridge Trail	F only	E	1.8	L	11	93
Volunteer Trail	F only	M	2.2	M to L	11	94
NATURE STATION TRAILS						
Center Furnace Trail	F only	E	0.3	M to H	3	96
Hematite Trail	F only	E	2.2	M to H	3	97
Honker Trail	F only	E	4.5	M to H	3	99
Long Creek Trail	F, B, E	E	0.4	M to H	3	100
Nature Station Connector Trail	F only	M	4.8	M	3	101
Token Trail Spring Spur Trail	F only	E	0.5	L to M	3	103
Woodland Walk	F only	E	1.0	M to H	3	103
NORTH-SOUTH TRAIL (Subdivided)						
South Welcome to Ginger Creek Road	F	M	13.7	M	10, 8	108
Ginger Creek Road to Golden Pond	F, E	M	15.1	M	8, 6	110
Golden Pond to Duncan Bay	F, B	M to D	18.0	M	6, 4	113
Duncan Bay to North Welcome	F, B	M	13.2	M	4, 2	117
NORTH-SOUTH SPUR TRAILS						
Brier Rose Spring Spur Trail	F only	M	0.2	L	10	124
Brown Spring Spur Trail	F only	E	0.2	M	2	124

■ TABLE KEY ■

TYPE: F = Foot   B = Bicycle   E = Equestrian
DIFFICULTY: M = Moderate   D = Difficult   L = Low
LENGTH: = miles   **USE:** M = Moderate   H = High

LAND BETWEEN THE LAKES TRAIL TABLE						
	TYPE	DIFFICULTY	LENGTH	USE	MAP	PAGE
NORTH-SOUTH SPUR TRAILS *(continued)*						
Brush Arbor Camp Spur Trail	F only	M to D	0.8	L	6	124
Buzzard Wing Spring Spur Trail	F only	E	0.1	L	4	125
Coffin Cove Spur Trail	F only	E	0.2	L	4	126
Colson Overlook Spur Trail	F only	M	0.4	L	6	126
Dead Beaver Spring Spur Trail	F only	M	0.8	L	4	127
Fort Henry Trail Connector	F only	E	1.4	M	10	127
Ferry Landing Spur Trail	F only	E	1.0	L	2	128
Golden Pond Spur Trail	F only	E	0.2	M	6	129
Jenny Ridge Spur Trail	F only	E	0.2	M	6	129
Laura Furnace Fork Spur Trail	F only	M	1.6	L	6	129
Model Loop Trail	F only	M	7.4	M	8	131
Mountain Laurel Spring Spur Trail	F only	M	0.8	L	6	134
Nightriders Spring Spur Trail	F only	E	0.6	M	2	135
Sugar Jack Spring Spur Trail	F only	M	1.0	L	4	136
Turkey Spring/School House Hollow Spring Spur Trail	F only	M	0.6	L	6	136
Walker Line Trail	F only	M	2.8	L	8	137

■ TABLE KEY ■

TYPE: F = Foot   B = Bicycle   E = Equestrian
DIFFICULTY: M = Moderate   D = Difficult   L = Low
LENGTH: = miles   **USE:** M = Moderate   H = High

Favorite Sights and Scenes at LBL

LAND BETWEEN THE Lakes is full of beauty. However, beauty is in the eye of the beholder, as the saying goes. While one person might desire lakeside fishing, another might want to see a variety of wildflowers. Yet another might want to travel beneath a towering forest. After exploring the entire recreation area, here are some of my favorite sights.

■ Seeing the jonquils bloom at all the old homesites in March

■ Reeling in a smallmouth bass from Pisgah Bay

■ Coasting down the Kentucky Lake bluffs on Canal Loop Trail

- Stopping on the Canal Loop Trail and jumping in Lake Barkley
- Walking up Bear Creek Valley
- Fall hiking on the Central Hardwoods Scenic Trail
- Watching a sheep shearing at The Homeplace
- Listening to the owls hoot at the Nature Station
- Heading down Wienger Hollow on a horse
- Watching elk calves trail their mother at Elk & Bison Prairie
- Learning where the constellations are at the Golden Pond Planetarium
- Spending a cool spring night at Laura Furnace Trail Shelter
- Finding wildflowers on the Telegraph Trail
- Contemplating Civil War soldiers who once followed the Telegraph Trail
- Taking a bird walk at Golden Pond Visitor Center
- Picnicking at Jenny Ridge
- Cooking out over a campfire at Gatlin Point Campground
- Canoeing on Honker Lake
- Absorbing the fall colors around Cedar Pond
- Getting a view of the river batteries of Fort Donelson Battlefield
- Absorbing the solitude on the Tennessee Ridge Trail
- Riding a horse-drawn wagon among the hardwoods along Fords Bay
- Swimming at Energy Lake Beach
- Getting chilled by a late winter wind at Redd Hollow Lake Access
- Walking down Duncan Creek valley on the Nature Station Trail Connector
- Enjoying an evening with equestrians at Wranglers Camp
- Looking out on Honker Lake from the dam
- Seeing old homesites on the most northerly section of the North–South Trail
- Relaxing by Hematite Lake while hoping a bream takes the bait
- Sea kayaking the canal connecting Lake Barkley and Kentucky Lake
- Eating persimmons in late October
- Standing on the state line dividing Tennessee and Kentucky on the Walker Line Trail
- Road biking down Mulberry Flat Road
- Watching the sun set from my gravel bar campsite on Kentucky Lake

- Being amazed at all the blooming dogwood trees scattered in the woods
- Making a scenic drive overlooking Kentucky Lake
- Camping at Piney Campground after day hiking the Picket Loop
- Checking out the buffalo from the South Bison Range Picnic Area
- Enjoying the open meadows near Tharpe
- Watching the deer graze near Long Creek
- Considering the lives of the ironworkers along the Center Furnace Trail
- Fishing Bards Lake in a johnboat
- Contemplating the Great Western Iron Furnace

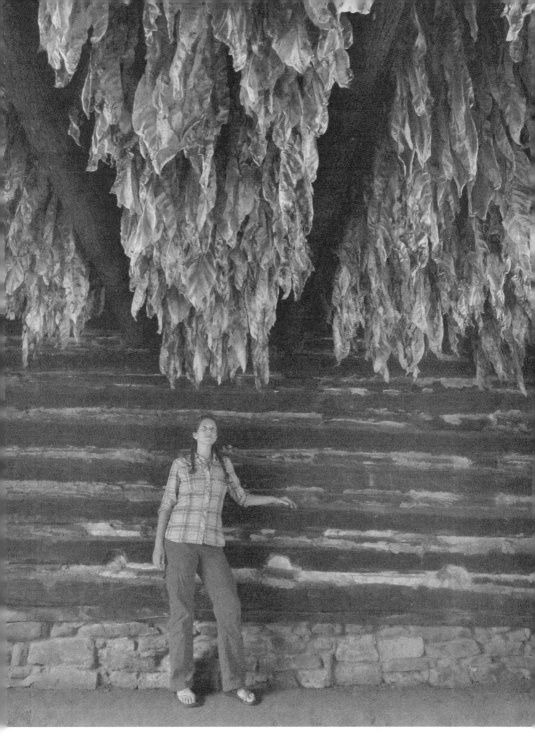

Handcut leaf hangs in the tobacco barn at The Homeplace.

PART ONE

• The Facilities •

Visitor Centers

■ GOLDEN POND VISITOR CENTER

NEAREST TOWN Canton, KY

OPEN Year-round, 9 a.m.–5 p.m.

FEES No

FACILITIES Restrooms, drinking water, telephone, human and natural history exhibits and videos, soft-drink machines, gift shop, picnic tables, grills, and playground

ACTIVITIES Viewing LBL exhibits and videos, seeing planetarium show, picnicking, hiking, road biking, mountain biking, nature study, and fishing

SERVICES Dispenses trail maps, information maps, fishing reports, and other recreation hand-outs; sells backcountry camping permits and entry cards for Elk & Bison Prairie, Woodlands Nature Station, The Homeplace; sells LBL- and area-related books, T-shirts, souvenirs, and Turkey Bay off-highway vehicle permits.

OTHER Visitor center is staffed with knowledgeable locals who will personally assist you with questions and information regarding your LBL experience.

GOLDEN POND VISITOR Center is the hub of LBL. It is centrally located at the recreation area and is at the junction of LBL's primary road, Woodlands Trace National Scenic Byway, and LBL's only east–west crossroad, US 68/KY 80. The recreation area administration offices and law enforcement center are here too. It makes sense to locate the main visitor center here.

Enter the visitor center and the LBL staff will be waiting to greet you and answer your questions. Inside are exhibits displaying the human and natural history of LBL. I highly recommend taking the time to read and look over the photographs, maps, and artifacts of the exhibits, including a video detailing the 50th anniversary of LBL. LBL's history lends a new perspective to this preserve. Also inside is the planetarium theater, where multimedia shows about the heavens above are held. The gift shop is located near the planetarium.

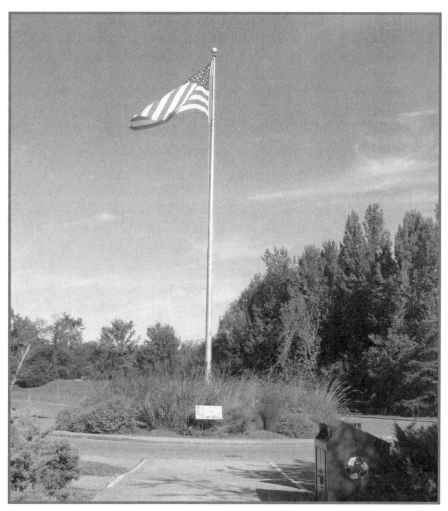

Golden Pond Visitor Center

The visitor center is attractively landscaped and has two ponds on site. A shaded picnic area and pavilion overlook one of the ponds toward the back of the visitor center. This pond is open to bank fishing. Hikers take note that the 1.4-mile Admin Loop leaves from here (see "Suggested Loops," pages 141–142). The Golden Pond Spur Trail leaves the visitor center and connects to the North–South Trail. Hiking on the North–South Trail is limited only by time. Hikers and bikers can enjoy the cross-peninsula Central Hardwoods Scenic Trail. The northbound portion of the North–South Trail is open to mountain bikes. Road bikers can head north or south on Woodlands Trace for a scenic pedal.

ACCESS Golden Pond Visitor Center is centrally located at LBL. It can be reached from the east and I-24 at Exit 65 via US 68/KY 80, from the north on I-24 from Exit 31 via KY 453 South, from the west by KY 80, and from the south by US 79 and Woodlands Trace.

■ NORTH WELCOME STATION

NEAREST TOWN Grand Rivers, KY

OPEN March–November, 9 a.m.–5 p.m. daily

FEES No

FACILITIES Restrooms, drinking water, telephone, soft-drink machine, picnic tables and grills, playground, dump station, and gift shop

ACTIVITIES Scenic driving, picnicking, hiking, and mountain and road biking

SERVICES Dispenses trail maps, information maps, and other recreation handouts; sells backcountry camping permits and entry cards for Elk & Bison Prairie, Woodlands Nature Station, The Homeplace; sells LBL- and area-related books, T-shirts, and souvenirs, and Turkey Bay off-highway vehicle permits.

OTHER Visitor center is manned with local, knowledgeable staff who will personally assist you with questions and information regarding your LBL experience.

MOST VISITORS ENTER Land Between The Lakes from the north end. Thus, the North Welcome Station is the more visited of the two welcome stations. Picnic tables and a playground offer a chance to get out of the car and relax before heading on to other LBL destinations. Conveniently located just 7 miles from I-24, this welcome station is a jumping-off point for many activities. Hikers and bikers use it as a trailhead for the Canal Loop trail system and the North–South Trail. The North End Hike/Bike Trail leaves from here and heads south for 1.5 miles to Hillman Ferry Campground, one of LBL's most popular overnighting locales. Cravens Bay is the other nearby campground. Road bikers will take off, heading south down Woodlands Trace National Scenic Byway.

Auto tourists will also head down Woodlands Trace. Kentucky Lake Scenic Drive is just north of the welcome center. Elevated vista points offer far-reaching views of Kentucky Dam to the north and the seemingly endless lake to the south. Nearby, Moss Creek Day-Use Area offers a swimming beach for the summer months. Those wanting to get on either Kentucky Lake or Lake Barkley have three nearby boat launches from which to choose.

ACCESS From Exit 31 on I-24 near Lake City, head south on KY 453 for 7 miles. Kentucky 453 becomes Woodlands Trace once it enters Land Between The Lakes National Recreation Area. The North Welcome Station will be on your right.

■ SOUTH WELCOME STATION

NEAREST TOWN Dover, TN

OPEN March–November, 9 a.m.–5 p.m. daily

FEES No

FACILITIES Restrooms, drinking water, telephone, soft-drink machine, picnic tables and grills, playground, dump station, and gift shop

ACTIVITIES Scenic driving, picnicking, hiking, and biking

SERVICES Dispenses trail maps, information maps, and other recreation handouts; sells backcountry camping permits and entry cards for Elk & Bison Prairie, Woodlands Nature Station, The Homeplace; sells LBL- and area-related books, T-shirts, and souvenirs, and Turkey Bay off-highway vehicle permits.

OTHER Visitor center is staffed with knowledgeable locals who will personally assist you with questions and information regarding your LBL experience.

THE SOUTH WELCOME Station is the first stop for those arriving at LBL from the Tennessee side of the recreation area. Visitors can get oriented here or simply start enjoying LBL. The helpful staff offers not only specific information about LBL points of interest, but also has handouts and information about neighboring parks and area tourist attractions.

Jumping right into LBL is easy, since the North–South Trail departs from here and runs 60-plus miles to reach the North Welcome Station. It also runs into a connector trail that joins the Fort Henry trail system to form the 6.6-mile Bear Creek Loop hike. If you want to see some of LBL by car, you can take the Woodlands Trace Scenic Drive or the South Loop Forest Drive, detailed in this book (see pages 151–154). Picnic tables are located behind the visitor center and across Woodlands Trace. Bicyclers will be seen unloading their two-wheelers to ply the Woodlands Trace or Fort Henry Road. Piney is the nearest fully developed campground, whereas Gatlin Point offers more primitive camping facilities.

ACCESS From Dover, TN, head south on US 79 for 5.0 miles to access Woodlands Trace. Turn right on Woodlands Trace and drive north for 3.4 miles to reach the welcome station on your right.

Visitor Facilities

■ SOUTH BISON RANGE

NEAREST TOWN Dover, TN
OPEN Year-round
FEES No
FACILITIES Picnic area and trail encircling range
ACTIVITIES Wildlife and nature study
OTHER South Bison Range can be enjoyed from vehicle on Woodlands Trace.

THE SOUTH BISON Range is home of the southern herd of LBL's buffalo, the original herd that lives on two adjacent 100-acre meadows. Introduced in 1969 shortly after the establishment of LBL, these bison came from North Dakota and, since they arrived, have enjoyed the grassy fields where the town of Model, Tennessee, once stood.

Buffalo once ranged over most of North America, including the land between the Cumberland and Tennessee Rivers. When white settlers first came into Tennessee and Kentucky, they often followed buffalo paths, which they called "traces." Perhaps this is how LBL's main road, Woodlands Trace, received its name.

A wide pulloff along Woodlands Trace allows observation of the buffalo, which can reach up to 2,000 pounds. Also included is an informative signboard. For a closer glimpse, hikers can see America's largest land animal via the Model Loop Trail, portions of which go directly alongside the fence separating you from these large, shaggy creatures. The Model Loop Trail begins at The Homeplace trailhead, just north of the South Bison Range.

Picnickers can dine at South Bison Range Picnic Area while they watch buffalo feed on the grasses. This picnic area is located on Woodlands Trace just across from the South Bison Range. A cross trail bisecting the South Bison Range is 0.2 mile south of the picnic area. Look for the wooden bridge over Prior Creek.

ACCESS From the South Welcome Station, head north on Woodlands Trace for 10 miles to the South Bison Range, on your left.

■ ELK & BISON PRAIRIE

NEAREST TOWN Grand Rivers, KY

OPEN Year-round, dawn–dusk

FEES Yes

FACILITIES None

ACTIVITIES Wildlife and nature study

OTHER Entrance to the prairie is cash/credit card–machine operated. Entrance cards can be purchased on site or at North Welcome Station, South Welcome Station, or Golden Pond Visitor Center.

THE ELK & Bison Prairie provides an opportunity for visitors to see these large animals in their native environment. The 3-plus-mile loop drive circles a 750-acre meadow mixed with woodland. Three informative stops along the drive avail more insight into this prairie ecosystem that has virtually disappeared from Kentucky. Only enclosed vehicles are allowed here. Motorcyclists, pedestrians, and bicyclers are prohibited from using the loop road. You can get out of your car inside the prairie, but if the animals are within 200 feet, do not get out of your car! These elk and bison are wild animals, hence unpredictable. Bison can run at speeds up to 35 miles an hour! In

Soaking in the interpretive information at the Elk & Bison Prairie

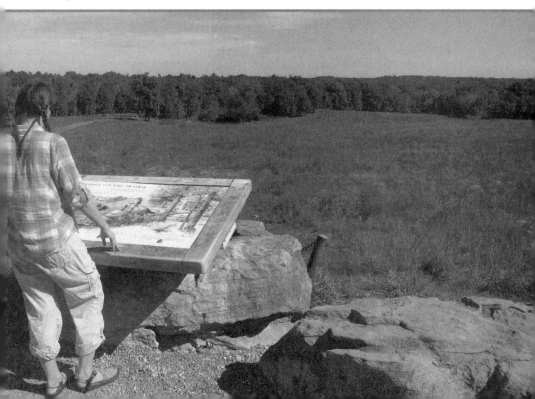

addition, once inside the prairie, you can drive the loop as many times as you want. Hiking is not allowed inside the prairie.

More than 200 years ago, much of western Kentucky was grassland. Periodic fires, primarily started by American Indians—Shawnee, Chickasaw, and Cherokee—established this grassland in order to attract the elk and bison for hunting. Herds of these animals would be lured to these grasslands, further keeping them open. The first area settlers called the prairies "barrens," because they were barren of trees. The Barren River, east of LBL, was named for these prairies. Settlers mistakenly thought the soil was too poor to support tree life. The forest soon reclaimed its place without the periodic burning, and settlers made their own clearings for cropland.

In these prairies, Indians would hunt elk and bison for meat, shelter, and tools. Tools were carved from bone; hides were made into tents, canoes, and moccasin soles. These animals were a veritable store on hooves. Of course, it took much work to transform the raw materials into usable goods.

Back in the 1970s, LBL biologists noticed patches of native grasses growing in portions of what is now the Elk & Bison Prairie. They began a program of controlled burns, expanding the clearings, causing the native grasses to return in grand fashion. The biologists then decided to add other elements of the prairie land—elk, bison, and additional native grasses. The prairie today is much like that of two or more centuries ago, when bison ranged from Florida to northern Canada and from the Appalachians to the Rockies.

Look for not only wildlife but also their signs, such as buffalo wallows, where the shaggy creatures cool off and get relief from bugs. Animal tracks, paths, and droppings are visible in the prairie. Enjoy the stops that offer interpretive information about the people, plants, and wildlife of the prairie. The rolling hills of grass broken with woodland make for scenic driving.

Nature photographers will be snapping pictures here in the upper valley of Crooked Creek. Each season offers its own perspective of the prairie. In spring, visitors will see the prairie after periodic burnings. Bison and elk calves will appear in late spring. During summer, the native prairie grasses grow high and wildlife keep to the cooler shadows. Try to visit the prairie early in the morning or late in the day during this time. Elk will be bugling—making their mating calls—in fall, and rubbing the velvet from their antlers. Winter can be the best time to view wildlife, as the leaves are off the trees and the animals will be feeding on clear, cold days.

Group rates are available for vans and buses. Information, restrooms, and water are available at the Golden Pond Visitor Center, located just south of the Elk & Bison Prairie on Woodlands Trace.

ACCESS From the entrance of Golden Pond Visitor Center, head north on Woodlands Trace for 0.9 mile. The Elk & Bison Prairie will be on your right.

■ THE HOMEPLACE

NEAREST TOWN Dover, TN
OPEN March and November, Wednesday–Saturday; April–October, open 7 days per week. Hours: Daily 10 a.m.–5 p.m.
FEES Yes, fee for ages 13 and up, lower fee for kids 5–12, free for ages 4 and under
FACILITIES Restrooms, water fountain, soft-drink machines, gift shop
ACTIVITIES Visit living history homestead with period interpreters acting out lives of the past.
OTHER The Homeplace can be enjoyed again and again through the seasons.

THE HOMEPLACE IS just one more unique offering of Land Between The Lakes. This is a living homestead, a place where interpreters, dressed in period clothing, go about the daily chores and activities typical of an 1850s northwest Tennessee farm. You've probably been places where old log buildings could be toured—the buildings at The Homeplace are authentic historic structures obtained from the LBL area. At LBL, the interpreters are on-site, adding life to the historic structures. The interpreters will be doing whatever the farmers would've been doing at that time:

Double Pen House at The Homeplace

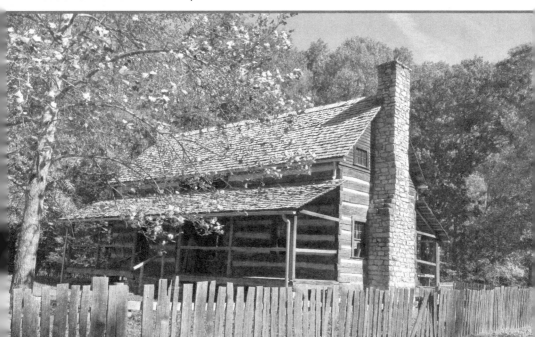

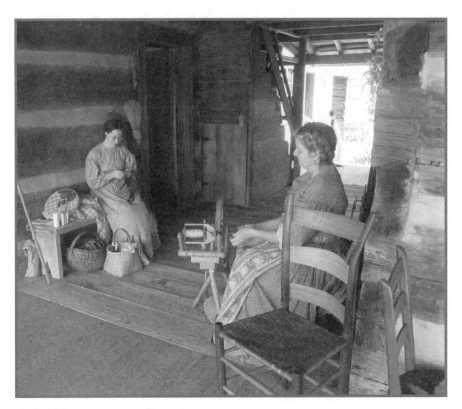

Period interpreters at The Homeplace

they may be plowing in spring, or hand carving a child's wooden toy by the fire in winter, using the spinning yarn, or tending the farm animals. Furthermore, while at The Homeplace, you are encouraged to interact with the interpreters, ask them questions about what they are doing and their daily lives, and lend a hand with the chores.

Enter the Interpretive Center, built into the ground as an energy-saving experiment by the Tennessee Valley Authority. Exhibits inside the center give you a taste of what is to come. Leave the center, pass a field, and enter the homestead. The sounds and smells of a real farm come alive. The double-pen house is always active with sewing, cooking, and additional household activities. The furnishings are period, too, enhancing the atmosphere. In summer, the nearby vegetable garden will be thriving. No chemicals are used here—only natural "fertilizer" from the livestock. The period accuracy extends even to the breeds of domestic critters on the farm. You'll see chickens, oxen, mules, and pigs.

A total of 16 structures can be explored. Look at the detail, down to the notched logs and square-head nails. Check out the tools hanging on the barn walls that farmers of that day used. Interpreters may very well be using them. Look inside the single-pen house and imagine living here day after day. Smell inside the smokehouse, where meat was cured for preservation. See the springhouse—the farm's refrigerator. Take your time and plan to come back, since the presentation changes with the seasons. The Homeplace also has special events every weekend beyond their daily activities. These events take a closer look at the foods, firearms, tools, and cultural aspects of the times. Check the LBL website for more information.

ACCESS From the South Welcome Station, take Woodlands Trace 10.6 miles north to The Homeplace.

■ GOLDEN POND PLANETARIUM

NEAREST TOWN Canton, KY
OPEN Daily 10 a.m.–5 p.m., closed Thanksgiving Day and Christmas Day through New Year's Day. Varied shows begin hourly on the hour starting at 10 a.m.; last show at 4 p.m. Additional evening shows on select dates.
FEES Yes, fee for ages 13 and up, lower fee for ages 5–12, free for ages 4 and under
FACILITIES 81-seat dome theater with multimedia presentation focusing on astronomy; qualified interpreters supplement presentations and interact with audience
ACTIVITIES Viewing presentation of varying programs
SERVICES Groups can schedule shows at other times and receive group rates.
OTHER The Golden Pond Planetarium is located inside the Golden Pond Visitor Center.

LIKE OTHER SPECIAL activities at Land Between The Lakes, the planetarium does not disappoint. For many LBL visitors, this is their first activity, since the planetarium is located inside the main visitor center. The planetarium offers rotating shows led by an avid astronomer who adds a human touch to the presentation. The theater has steeply sloped seating from which you look upon a domed screening area, where presentations are made. The shows here rival planetariums in any big city. After the primary show, the astronomer projects onto the dome what the local skies will look like that night, no matter the time of year. He will then point out stars, constellations, and other interesting features of the night sky that will leave you wishing for sunset to hurry up and come.

This is not just a presentation for school kids, though school groups would certainly enjoy the presentation. Additionally, the shows do correlate with Tennessee and Kentucky educational standards. It is something that everyone, including adults, can enjoy. It certainly opened my eyes to worlds far beyond our own and was worth the small expense and the hour of my time.

An observatory, located behind the visitor center, is open periodically for "Star Parties" and public observation sessions, led by local astronomers. For current planetarium shows and observatory events, consult the LBL website.

ACCESS The Golden Pond Planetarium is located inside the Golden Pond Visitor Center. It can be reached from the east on I-24 at Exit 65 via US 68/KY 80, from the north on I-24 from Exit 31 via KY 453 South, from the west by KY 80, and from the south by US 79 and Woodlands Trace.

■ WOODLANDS NATURE STATION

NEAREST TOWN Canton, KY
OPEN March and November, Wednesday–Sunday; April–October, 7 days per week. Hours: 10 a.m.–5 p.m. Closed Thanksgiving Day and December through February
FEES Yes, fee for ages 13 and up, lower fee for ages 5–12, free for ages 4 and under
FACILITIES Restrooms, water fountain, soft-drink machines, gift shop
ACTIVITIES Animal and nature study
OTHER Nature Station has on-site naturalists who enhance the experience.

COMMONLY REFERRED TO simply as the "Nature Station," the Woodlands Nature Station offers an opportunity to see the animals of Land Between The Lakes up close. Upon visiting, I feared some hokey exhibit, but found the experience offered much more. I encourage all those interested in wildlife to see the Nature Station for themselves. It is the gateway for the 8,500-acre Nature Watch Area.

Enter the Learning Center. Here, turtles, snakes, and other amphibians of LBL reside. Down low, for the kids, are hands-on displays, where they can feel the different pelts of animals and compare the different skull shapes and sizes. Another area features a beaver pond exhibit with a touch table.

Enter the Backyard Exhibit Area, an attractive area housing numerous birds and land animals. It is also landscaped with native plants and gardens to attract hummingbirds and butterflies. Take a walk around and see the animals. The Backyard Exhibit Area is the one and only refuge for these nonreleasable critters that were injured, orphaned, or born in captivity. Most often when seeing wildlife in the wild, all we see is the tail end of the critter running into a thicket. Here visitors can see and study these animals up close. To see their facial expressions and nuances of movement is truly fascinating. The

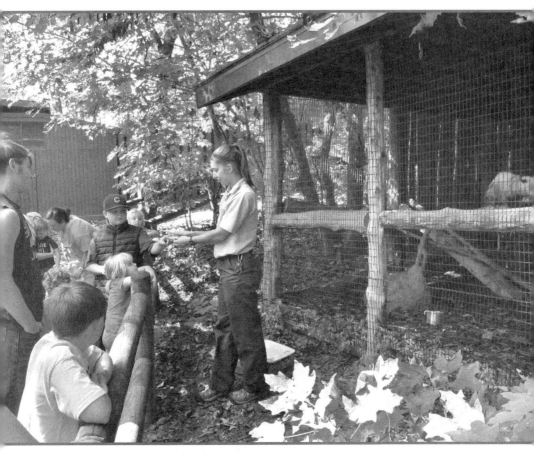

Naturalists hold daily programs at the Nature Station.

pens are large and offer freedom of movement. Furthermore, the on-site naturalists are there to answer your questions and will lead groups through the Backyard Exhibit Area. They put together nature's puzzle, informing visitors about the interrelationships between plants and animals at Land Between The Lakes.

See a bald eagle, white-tailed deer, vultures, and wild turkeys. The bald eagle oozes majesty when viewed this close. One pond is stocked with fish native to the area. Another pond is for turtles. Yet another pond has many of the smaller life-forms found in a wetland. The Nature Station has the only red wolves in Kentucky. Particularly enjoyable was what I call "Raptor Row." Here, side by side, are a red-tailed hawk, American kestrel, great horned owl, barred owl, screech owl, and barn owl. You can see and compare them and, if you are lucky, hear and learn each one's unique call.

Animal feedings are a daily event and times are posted. Stick around if you can. Special events and seasonal programs are held throughout the year. Naturalists lead hikes, eagle-watching tours, popular canoe trips in Honker Lake, and walking "creek crawls." Naturalists also seek wildlife at night and lead van tours of particular LBL locales. Call ahead at 270-924-2299 to find out which animals, insects, plants, or habitat are featured on the day of your visit and what times they will occur. The Parade of Raptors is held daily at 4:30 p.m.

Canoes can be rented daily between Memorial Day and Labor Day for nonguided paddle trips on Honker Lake. School and youth groups are welcome at the Nature

Turtles at the Nature Station

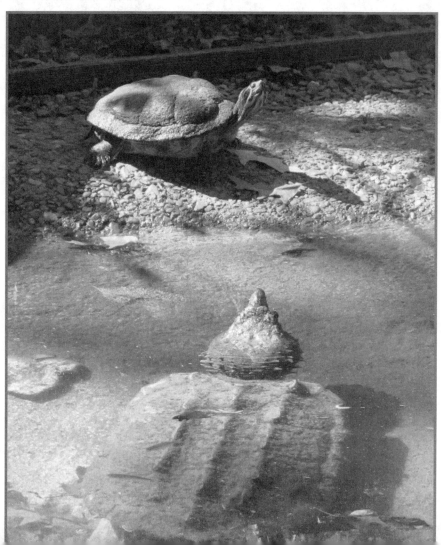

NATURE WATCH AREAS

LBL, since its establishment, has been a haven of flora and fauna. Thus, it is no surprise that this national recreation area has become popular for viewing nature's finest spectacles, from wildflowers to wildlife. Nature study has grown in popularity, and LBL is poised to accommodate this phenomenon, starting with the Nature Station, where visitors can consult with professional naturalists, learning where to see bald eagles, hear frogs croak, and smell blooming lotus. To enhance visitor opportunities, LBL has established two Nature Watch Areas, so visitors can focus on the best nature-watching spots.

The Woodlands Nature Watch Area is LBL's largest nature watch area at 6,800 areas, with the Nature Station in its center. The Woodlands Nature Watch Area encompasses what once was the Kentucky Woodlands National Wildlife Refuge, a predecessor to LBL. Here, bottomlands, fields, forests, and wetlands—as well as freshwater impounds such as Hematite Lake, Honker Lake, and Energy Lake—increase biodiversity. Nature enthusiasts have multiple ways to view fauna such as beaver, waterfowl, wild turkeys, otters, and osprey, as well as flora such as blooming bushes and brilliantly colored trees. Nature lovers can see this flora and fauna in a number of ways: drive roads, hike trails, and paddle waters.

The Southern Nature Watch Area lies in Tennessee, near the Fort Henry area. Coming in at 1,400 acres, it boasts LBL's most productive wildflower locale. Here, upland hills and rock outcrops, combined with a mature forest heavy with beech and maple, make the Southern Nature Watch Area excellent for fall color viewing too.

Winter eagle watching is one of LBL's biggest wildlife watch draws. Wildflowers in spring bring visitors in as well. To know what nature to see in every season, consult the experts at the Nature Station, and make the most of these specially designated nature watch areas.

Station. Reservations are encouraged in order to give each group time and space at the Nature Station. Call the above number for more information.

ACCESS From the entrance of Golden Pond Visitor Center, head north on Woodlands Trace for 9.2 miles to Silver Trail Road, FR 133. Turn right on Silver Trail Road and follow it for 3.1 miles to dead-end at the Woodlands Nature Station.

PART TWO

▪ The Lakes ▪

Boating

IT COMES AS NO SURPRISE THAT boating is popular at Land Between The Lakes National Recreation Area. Consider the reasons why: LBL is encircled by water on three sides, forming over 300 miles of winding shoreline on its boundaries. LBL has over a dozen lake access areas, plus other boat launches at its campgrounds. In addition to the two big lakes—Kentucky Lake and Lake Barkley—it has five other lakes suitable for boating. Boating opportunities range from powering up the wide Kentucky Lake in a cabin cruiser to paddling a canoe on quiet Duncan Lake. LBL visitors motorboat for pleasure, simply enjoying the scenic islands of Lake Barkley in a houseboat or while pulling a skier behind a speedboat. Others will be using a bass boat in pursuit of fish. There will be yachts tooling in the Tennessee River channel and johnboats putting in and out of small bays. Still others will be paddling smaller craft. Canoeing has always been popular on the smaller subimpoundments of LBL, such as Honker Lake, and more and more paddlers are exploring the big lakes. Sea kayakers have discovered the possibilities of paddling LBL. Sea kayaks, stable in waves and sleek in a wind, are plying the big lakes along the LBL shoreline, offering to paddlers wildlife viewing, fishing, and camping. So no matter your craft of choice, find a boat launch and enjoy this watery paradise.

Maps of both Kentucky Lake and Lake Barkley are available on the Internet at **kentuckylake.com,** a site loaded with information of interest to area boaters.

MOTORBOATING

ANY VISITOR TO LAND BETWEEN THE LAKES will undoubtedly see an auto with a boat and trailer in tow. They are heading for the numerous boat launches at the individual recreation areas. Fishing boats more often head for the lake access launches and pleasure boats often use the campground launches. The two big lakes, Barkley and Kentucky, are open to any type of craft, including tug-pushed barges filled with products. Watch out for these massive craft. Other smaller lakes in LBL have horse-power and motor limitations. See the subsequent fishing section for boating rules if you plan to ply a smaller lake. All boaters must meet boating regulations concerning life jackets and registration for the state in which they are boating.

CANOEING AND KAYAKING

ENERGY LAKE AND HONKER LAKE are the most popular places for canoeing and light kayaking at Land Between The Lakes. Both of these impoundments have rental boats on-site during the warm season. This arrangement offers paddling opportunities for those who don't own their own boats. Paddlers will find that wildlife sightings are much more likely when you are exploring waters in a quiet canoe rather than in a motorboat. However, the going is much slower. Hematite Lake and Bards Lake, sub-impoundments of Lake Barkley, are also good for paddling.

As paddling has grown in popularity, paddlers have discovered the many bays of both Kentucky Lake and Lake Barkley. The bays of Kentucky Lake are deeper and larger than Barkley's bays, offering shelter from the winds that can blow down the main lake while allowing plenty of room for exploration. Paddlers on Kentucky Lake should consider Ginger Bay, Sugar Bay, and Smith Bay, which all have conventional boat launches. Pisgah Bay is also good but can be busy with motorboat anglers. More adventurous paddlers will get an LBL downloadable map and take secondary roads

Kayak awaits on KY Lake.

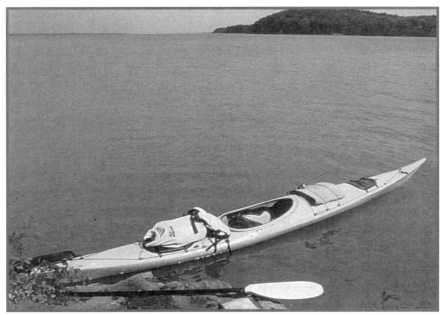

to reach more remote bays, like Hughes Bay, Clay Bay, and Barnett Bay. Be careful on those back roads; they can become rutted and muddy.

The bays of Lake Barkley are generally smaller than Kentucky Lake's. Neville Bay offers a conventional boat launch. Devils Elbow Boat Launch has a small pond-like area between US 68 and the old US 68 roadbed, keeping down wind and waves. Car noise detracts from the setting, however. Long Creek Pond, just across US 68 from Devils Elbow, is a scenic body of water, but is also subject to auto noise. Lake Barkley does have some excellent remote bays accessible by back roads. Consider paddling Mammoth Furnace Bay, Carmack Bay, Crockett Bay, and Prior Bay. Overall, paddlers are limited only by time and desire and could circumnavigate LBL on a several-day trip on the LBL Paddle Route below.

SEA KAYAKING

THE WINDING SHORELINE of the big lakes, broken by many bays, makes for ideal sea kayaking waters. Having lower profile boats, sea kayakers will be able to explore the big lakes with more ease than canoers. And with a backcountry camping permit, extended overnight trips along the shores of Land Between The Lakes can be undertaken. What makes camping even better is the option of overnighting on a rustic shoreline or taking advantage of more developed campgrounds such as Hillman Ferry or Cravens Bay. You could even consider mixing up backcountry and developed campgrounds.

LAND BETWEEN THE LAKES PADDLE ROUTE

LOOK AT A MAP OF THE UNITED STATES, then focus on middle America. Try to find any body of water with 300 miles of undeveloped shoreline, and you'll find only one—Land Between The Lakes. Here, paddlers in both canoes and sea kayaks can travel along the bays and bluffs of Kentucky Lake and Lake Barkley. Adventurous paddlers can circumnavigate the long peninsula of LBL, nearly making a loop, with the departure and arrival points separated by less than 10 miles of land. This way, paddlers can go for days without backtracking and still end up fairly close to their car and point of origin. The 85-mile paddle route is the shortest possible route of an LBL peninsula circumnaviga-tion, without exploring bays or making any side trips. A look at the map will show that this route can be extended by many miles and from five days to over two weeks.

This circumnavigation of the LBL peninsula is what I call the Land Between The Lakes Paddle Route, the best paddling area in middle America. The route begins on Kentucky Lake at Boswell Landing Lake Access in Tennessee. Paddlers then head north along Kentucky Lake, passing numerous large bays along the way to the

Kentucky state line. Lake accesses and campgrounds occasionally break wild shore-line. Kentucky Dam eventually comes into view. Here, paddlers take Barkley Canal joining Kentucky Lake to Lake Barkley.

Paddlers leave the canal, heading east, past Kuttawa Landing Lake Access. Beyond here, Lake Barkley turns south and paddlers pass the largest bays of Barkley. Islands appear more frequently south of the US 68/KY 80 bridge. Finally, paddlers reenter the Volunteer State and end the paddle route at the boat launch near Gatlin Point Campground. From here, it is but 10 miles by road to Boswell Landing.

Kentucky Lake

THE LBL PADDLE ROUTE is broken into two segments, Kentucky Lake and Lake Barkley. This first segment begins at Boswell Landing and travels north for 35 miles along the northernmost end of Kentucky Lake. Add one more mile passing through the Barkley Canal, the canal connecting Kentucky Lake and Lake Barkley. Boswell Landing makes for a good getaway spot, with its courtesy dock and boat ramp. From

Kentucky Lake

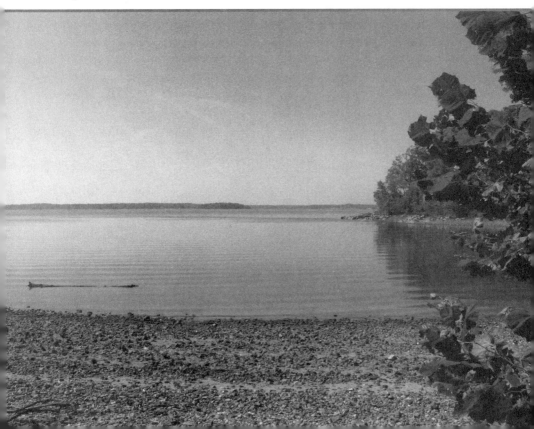

here paddlers can see far north up Kentucky Lake. Upon entering the water, paddlers will be surprised at the width of the lake, easily a mile wide. This width can cause problems if big winds kick up. However, the biggest surprise may be the changing character of the wild shoreline—hilly, tree-covered banks; rock bluffs; clay bluffs; and gravel bars all melded into a winding border between water and land.

And there is so much shoreline to explore—deep bays with numerous arms leading up quiet coves cutting deep into the heart of LBL beg to be paddled. On the main lake, civilization is barely visible across the water. Occasional giant barge loads pushed by low-humming tugs ply the old bed of the Tennessee River channel. Pleasure boaters and fishing boats will be seen, especially on weekends.

Pine Bluff stands far above the lake 5 miles north of Boswell Landing. Ginger Bay Lake Access lies 2 miles north of the bluff. No services are offered at either location. The gravel bars on the main shoreline, where the landings are easy, are your best bet for camping on Kentucky Lake. Rushing Creek flows into in a small cove on the main shore 10 miles north of Boswell. Enter Kentucky just beyond Rushing Creek. A large shoreline sign marks the state boundary. Anglers must have a fishing license for each state in which they are fishing.

Redd Hollow Lake Access lies in a cove 2 miles north of the state line, where Kentucky Lake narrows a bit. Beyond here the Eggners Ferry Bridge becomes visible. Fenton Campground, with potable water, is on the LBL shoreline just before the bridge. Kenlake State Park is on the western shore by the bridge. The lake widens again north of the bridge. Deeply cut bays are interspersed along the main shoreline here. Exploration opportunities are numerous along this wild shore, and the rocky point just south of Higgins Bay makes for a good breaking spot.

Things become more developed farther north. Smith Bay, part of Birmingham Ferry Campground, 28 miles north of Boswell, marks the beginning of this developed area. Just ahead is large Hillman Ferry Campground, which offers potable water and hot showers. The north end of the campground is closer to the main lake channel. Twin Lakes Lake Access and Moss Creek Day-Use Area come next. By now, the Kentucky Dam may be visible. Pass high bluffs then metal pillars used to steady barges just before reaching the Barkley Canal, 35 miles north of Boswell Landing. Pass through the rock-lined watery connector and keep along the LBL shoreline. Paddlers may experience a strong current here. Which way this current flows depends on which watershed—the Tennessee River or the Cumberland River—has received more rainfall recently. Barkley Dam is visible to your left after passing through the canal. Ahead on your right is Nickell Branch Lake Access and the end of the Kentucky Lake section.

Lake Barkley

THE SECOND PORTION of the LBL Paddle Route is longer—50 miles, and that is traveling the shortest route possible with no side tripping. Lake Barkley is narrower than Kentucky Lake. Long, slender islands break Barkley's lower part, potentially causing navigational problems. Getting around Kentucky Lake is simpler; head north and keep the LBL shoreline to your right. Barkley's shoreline is well forested with few gravel bars and few bluffs. The densely forested banks make finding a backcountry campsite challenging. Scout around the mouths of streams entering the lake—they tend to offer more level ground. Be prepared to search for a suitable campsite. However, the numerous lake accesses on Barkley can always function as backup campsites. The old Cumberland River channel swings all over Lake Barkley. Barges and bigger boats often follow this channel, as Barkley is riddled with shallows (which normally don't affect smaller propelled boats). It is important to check the lake level of Lake Barkley before paddling here.

Lake Barkley

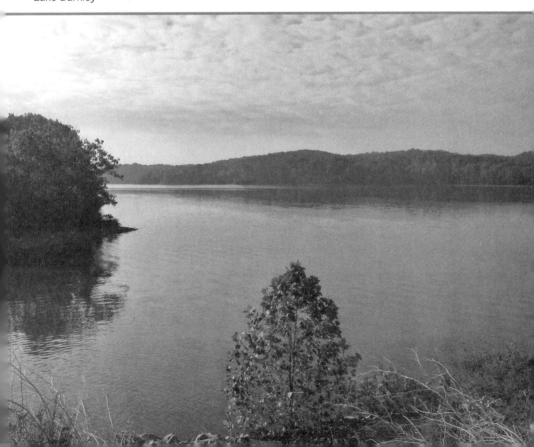

Begin this segment at Nickell Branch Lake Access and work east along the northern end of LBL. Large bays, like Demumbers Bay, characterize this area. Younger trees on the shoreline tell of a heavily settled area returning to forest. Curve north, coming to Kuttawa Lake Access at 8 miles. Beyond the landing, the paddle route turns south and stays southbound for the rest of the route, shortly passing Eddyville Ferry Lake Access in a hollow. Interestingly, the big building of the Kentucky State Penitentiary lies across the lake here. Look for the water tower with "KSP" inscribed on it.

Big bays cut into LBL below Kuttawa. A portion of Cravens Bay Campground stands on the main shoreline at 17 miles. Potable water can be had here. Ahead are the first islands and the Environmental Education (EE) Area. No camping is allowed in the EE Area, which is bordered on the north by Fulton Bay and on the south by part of Taylor Bay. Be aware that camping is allowed at Taylor Bay Lake Access at 23 miles.

Paddlers may want to consider entering Crooked Creek Bay. It offers good fishing and a developed campground on the far side of Energy Lake Dam. This would require a carry over the low dam. Keeping south on the now narrower main lake, reach the US 68/KY 80 bridge at 30 miles. Devils Elbow Lake Access is just south of here. The shoreline remains wild for more miles below Fords Bay ramp. Islands appear with regularity at this point. Smart paddlers will positively identify Neville Bay at 46 miles (you can see the grassy lake access from the main lake) and keep the LBL shoreline within view. Otherwise, you may miss the Gatlin Point Campground ramp and takeout, as several very long narrow islands block Gatlin Point from view if paddlers follow the main river channel. The Gatlin Point boat ramp, at 85 miles, marks the end of the LBL Paddle Route.

Fishing

THE TWO PRIMARY FISHING AREAS at Land Between The Lakes are the impoundments on either side of the recreation area: Kentucky Lake and Lake Barkley. The Tennessee Valley Authority created these impoundments decades apart, then cut a canal connecting them, thus creating the water boundaries of LBL.

The big lakes are not the only fisheries here. Several fishable ponds and lakes lie within the LBL borders. Some are old farm ponds; others are known as subimpoundments, which are smaller lakes separated from Lake Barkley by only a dam. Generally, these lakes offer species similar to the two big lakes: crappie, bass, catfish, and bream. Anglers must have a fishing license for the state in which they are fishing.

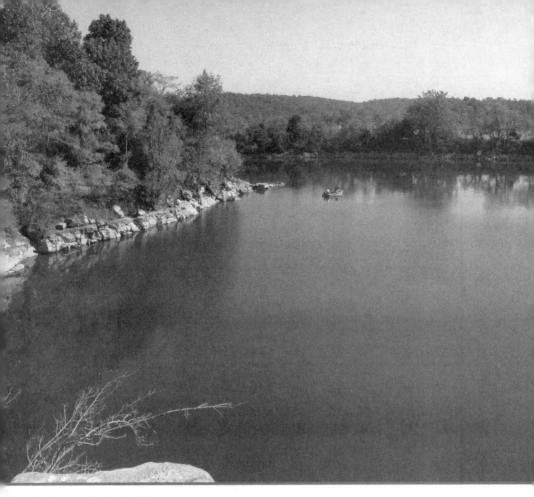

Anglers on Kentucky Lake

LBL is ringed with bait shops, marinas, and fishing-supply stores no matter your approach. Fishing licenses are available at these stores. The states of Kentucky and Tennessee both require a valid fishing license to angle in their waters.

Creel limits change year to year; for the latest limits contact either the Kentucky Department of Fish and Wildlife Resources or the Tennessee Wildlife Resources Agency.

FISHING REPORT

A GOOD RESOURCE FOR ANGLERS visiting Land Between The Lakes is **explore kentuckylake.com.** Here, you can access several fishing reports from guides operating on both Barkley and Kentucky Lakes.

LBL MONTH-TO-MONTH FISHING CHART				
	BASS	BREAM	CATFISH	CRAPPIE
JANUARY	Poor	Poor	Poor	Fair
FEBRUARY	Poor	Poor	Fair	Good
MARCH	Fair	Fair	Good	Excellent
APRIL	Good	Fair	Good	Excellent
MAY	Excellent	Excellent	Excellent	Excellent
JUNE	Good	Good	Excellent	Fair
JULY	Fair	Good	Excellent	Fair
AUGUST	Fair	Good	Good	Fair
SEPTEMBER	Good	Good	Good	Good
OCTOBER	Excellent	Good	Good	Excellent
NOVEMBER	Good	Fair	Fair	Good
DECEMBER	Fair	Poor	Fair	Fair

LAKE LEVELS

LAKE LEVELS AT KENTUCKY LAKE and Lake Barkley vary throughout the year. The two lakes are usually at the same level since a canal joins them. Water levels affect fishing, so it is advantageous to know average lake levels. For current lake levels visit **barkley.uslakes.info/Level** or **kentucky.uslakes.info/Level.** On the facing page is a diagram of month-to-month lake levels. Some day-to-day variations in water levels occur, but levels generally follow this graph. Floods or droughts will affect water levels.

KENTUCKY LAKE

FISHING ENTHUSIASTS FROM BOTH KENTUCKY AND TENNESSEE claim Kentucky Lake as their state's best big lake fishery. It is that good. And it is big enough for two states to stake a claim. From Kentucky Dam just north of LBL's northern end, Kentucky Lake stretches for a whopping 184 miles south, far into the Volunteer State. Kentucky Lake was impounded in the 1940s, as the Tennessee Valley Authority (TVA) sought to harness the floodwaters of the problematic Tennessee River, simultaneously making the river more reliable for water traffic and generating hydroelectric power. At the same time, TVA created what Arthur B. Lander Jr., in his book *A Fishing Guide to Kentucky's Major Lakes,* calls a "nationally recognized fishery," especially in terms of bass and crappie.

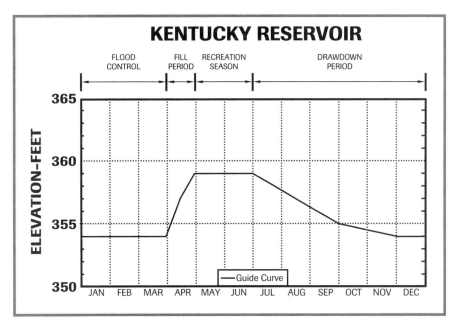

KENTUCKY RESERVOIR

| FLOOD CONTROL | FILL PERIOD | RECREATION SEASON | DRAWDOWN PERIOD |

Lake levels

Kentucky Lake seems to draw anglers no matter what the season. Spring has smallmouth bass and crappie anglers. The first warm days see smallmouth anglers on shallow bars at the mouths of creeks, throwing crank baits and jerk baits. But visitors will see more crappie anglers than any other in the season of rebirth. Brad Weakley, area fishing guide of over two decades, puts it this way, "These two lakes are known worldwide for crappie fishing. I have carried people from several different countries crappie fishing. You can catch crappie here in excess of three pounds. You don't get anybody's attention with a pound-and-a-half crappie on this lake." The prime crappie fishing will be between the 5th and 20th of April. When the redbuds are in full bloom and dogwoods are in bloom, the crappie will be spawning. Crappie can be caught in shallow water in good numbers using minnows.

Big bass fishing will pick up the beginning of May, when the largemouth will begin their prespawn feed. During this time, the spawn anglers go top water for ol' bucketmouth. Summertime anglers need to fish early and late for white bass using spinners or cast points with crank baits. Just find something else to do besides fish during midday. Smallmouth action picks up, especially using surface lures, when the first cool fronts blow through the region. The smallmouth bite can last into December if the weather is relatively warm.

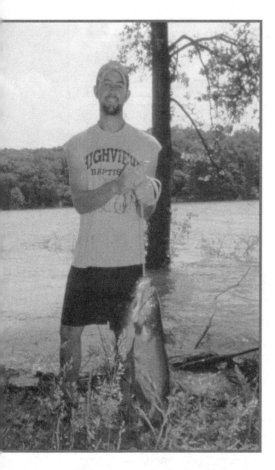

LBL angler proudly displays his catch.

In May, catfish anglers gather below Kentucky Dam in what is called "the world's largest catfish hole." Live (and not-so-live) bait is used in Kentucky Lake shallows during this time. In summer, anglers go deep and fish at night with chicken livers, stink baits, or even hot dogs. In September, folks go deep along the old Tennessee River channel for the big ones.

Bream begin their spawn in May. If you get on a bed, the numbers of fish caught can be staggering. However, bream fishing from lake access areas and banks can be good throughout the summer, making for great family fun. Use crickets, red worms, or wax worms, fished 3 to 4 feet deep, casting from the shore.

Winter is the quietest fishing time, but some anglers can still be seen fishing ledges for crappie and the old Tennessee River channel for sauger.

Of special note is the canal between Kentucky Lake and Lake Barkley. Oftentimes, the canal has a current, which is good for fishing. The direction of this current depends upon which watershed, the Cumberland River or Tennessee River, is pushing more water downstream. The current causes baitfish to move, and the predator fish follow them.

Hillman Ferry is a recommended angler base camp on Kentucky Lake. It is near Pisgah Bay, which is good for smallmouth, crappie, and white bass. Piney offers good angling opportunities too. All of the lake access areas are not bad bets.

LAKE BARKLEY

BARKLEY IS MUCH SMALLER and younger than Kentucky Lake. This impoundment of 60,000 acres was flooded in the 1960s. Barkley is also narrower and more crooked than Kentucky, allowing for fishing on windy days. If you encounter wind, consider fishing Barkley, which has far more wind-breaking islands than does

Kentucky Lake. Barkley, though, is more dangerous to run, with its numerous shallows. Brad Weakley advises anglers to "learn the channel buoys, you can run aground." (Remember the buoys: "red, right, return.")

Arthur Lander, in *A Fishing Guide to Kentucky's Major Lakes*, gives this overview: "Lake Barkley is a classic flatland reservoir with a wide variety of structure, from roadbeds, stump rows, and brush piles in shallow embayments to river channel islands, rock bluffs, and gravel points. There are some definite drop-offs along the old river channel, whereas on Kentucky Lake there are lots of gradually sloping points." A lot of water pushes through the narrow reservoir, making it a fertile lake. It generally follows the seasonal fishing patterns of Kentucky Lake.

Jerry Schwartz was a tournament angler from Indiana who simply fell in love with the lakes of LBL. He moved to the area and has been guiding other anglers ever since. Lake Barkley is his specialty. He recommends getting a lake map that details fishing "hot spots." These maps, which show depths and contour lines, as well as the hot spots, are generally available at any area tackle store. Next, go online and look up **kentuckylake.com** to find out the current water level and lake temperature (the website shows the water temperature of Lake Barkley as well). Wait until the water temperature is at least 50 degrees and preferably 55 degrees, then get out there and fish the main lake points for bass with crank baits and spinners. "This is your best chance for getting the big bass," Schwartz told me. "Go for crappie in coves around brush piles. Fish with minnows 4 to 5 feet deep in 10 to 12 feet of water. When the water temperature hits 60 degrees, the bass and crappie will pick up. The fish will be shallower. Drift across flats on the inner parts of bays."

Catfishing can be very good in May. Try the rock banks along the cliff wall south of Devils Elbow. Use leeches or night crawlers and a bobber, and drop your line down 3 to 4 feet deep. Arthur Lander recommends fishing the riprap (rock banks) on the old US 68 bridge at Devils Elbow Lake Access. Later in the summer, try at points where creek channels meet the main river channel.

Largemouth bass fishing can rival Kentucky Lake, but Lake Barkley doesn't have the numbers of smallmouth as does its sister lake to the west. Anglers see success on the embayments in the north end of LBL. White bass fishing can be very good in summer. Try the mouths of bays where the creeks drop off using a 3/8-ounce white rooster tail lure. Interestingly, when the dog days of summer hit, bass fishing can be better than you think. Dam operators start running water through the dams to generate electricity for air conditioning, and bass will be found along ledges and humps in the lake, chasing bait in the running currents.

Bream are also a favorite when the water temperature gets above 65 degrees. Head to the very back parts of bays, especially small coves or pockets. Bait a gold hook with crickets or mealworms. Bream will keep biting throughout the summer.

During fall, the bass follow the shad back into the bays from the main river. Try a Cordell crank bait in the Smoky Joe color, or 0.5-ounce spinner with willow leaf blades. Cast a jig tipped with a minnow for crappie in the bays.

Lake Barkley is the only lake in the two states that can give Kentucky Lake a run for its money on the crappie fishing. In fact, some anglers claim Lake Barkley is as good as Kentucky Lake. However, Barkley doesn't have the fishing pressure of Kentucky Lake.

Taylor Bay and Nickell Branch lake accesses are two of the more favored camps and jumping-off areas for Lake Barkley anglers. Jerry Schwartz likes Energy Lake Campground as an angling base camp. This area of Lake Barkley has crappie, bass, and bluegill in the immediate bays. "Some of the best LBL fishing on Barkley lies between Prior Bay on the state line to Taylor Bay," states Schwartz. One last tip: bank fish from the rocks below the bridge on FR 174 at Prior Bay.

OTHER FISHING LAKES, PONDS, AND STREAMS

■ BARDS LAKE

STATE Tennessee   **LAKE ACREAGE** 320 acres   **OPEN** Year-round
USE Low to moderate   **SPECIAL REGULATIONS** No-wake lake

BARDS LAKE IS a subimpoundment near the south end of LBL. A dam separates it from Lake Barkley. Brandon Springs Group Center borders part of the shoreline. Gatlin Point Campground offers easy access to the lake. Gasoline-powered engines are allowed on the lake, but at no-wake speeds.

ACCESS From the South Welcome Station, take Woodlands Trace north 0.9 mile to FR 227. Turn right on FR 227 and follow it 2.0 miles. Veer left on FR 229 and follow it 1.5 miles. Bards Lake is on the west side of the dam over which FR 229 leads.

■ CEDAR POND

STATE Tennessee   **LAKE ACREAGE** 2 acres   **OPEN** Year-round
USE Moderate   **SPECIAL REGULATIONS** No minnows

CEDAR POND, IN my opinion, is the most attractive body of water inside LBL. This old farm pond has a picnic area on its shore. A short gravel trail makes for easy access by bank anglers, and it's conveniently located beside Woodlands Trace.

ACCESS From the South Welcome Station, go north on Woodlands Trace 12.7 miles to the picnic area, on your right, just before the Tennessee–Kentucky state line.

■ DUNCAN LAKE

STATE Kentucky   **LAKE ACREAGE** 10 acres   **OPEN** March 16–October 31
USE Moderate to high   **SPECIAL REGULATIONS** No gas engines

LOCATED IN THE upper watershed of Duncan Creek, Duncan Lake is isolated from other impoundments. The pretty lake is known for bream fishing. Anglers can fish from the shore or launch their small boat from a grassy access area. Duncan Lake is closed during the winter months, as it is a waterfowl refuge.

ACCESS From Golden Pond Visitor Center, take Woodlands Trace north 9.3 miles to FR 132. Turn left on FR 132 and follow it 0.7 mile. Veer right on a gated gravel road leading downhill and follow it to a grassy flat beside Duncan Lake.

Duncan Lake

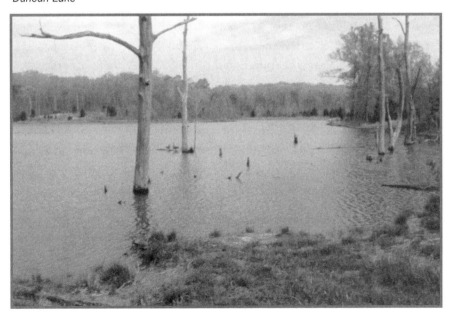

■ EDDYVILLE FERRY PONDS

STATE Kentucky   **LAKE ACREAGE** 1 acre each   **OPEN** Year-round
USE Low   **SPECIAL REGULATIONS** No minnows

THE EDDYVILLE FERRY PONDS are located off Old Ferry Road in the little-visited northeastern section of LBL. These are old farm ponds that offer a quiet fishing experience. The west-side pond is easily accessed from Old Ferry Road, whereas the east-side pond is off in the woods. The west-side pond is also easy to fish around. The east-side pond is wooded nearly all the way around its bank. These ponds are good for solitude, especially during the week.

ACCESS From the North Welcome Station, take Woodlands Trace south 5.3 miles to paved FR 117, Old Ferry Road. Turn left on FR 117 and follow it 6.2 miles. Look for the small pond to your left. The other pond is in the woods to your right.

■ ENERGY LAKE

STATE Kentucky   **LAKE ACREAGE** 370 acres
OPEN Year-round; except western third open March 16–October 31
USE High   **SPECIAL REGULATIONS** No-wake lake

ENERGY LAKE IS a popular fishing area. A boat ramp allows easy entry and exit at Energy Dam Lake Access Area. Campers can enjoy Energy Lake Campground. Boatless anglers can rent a canoe near the campground. Many anglers bank fish from the dam that divides Energy Lake from Lake Barkley. The western third of the lake is closed in winter, as it is a wildlife refuge. Summer can be noisy from the swim beach that is located on the shoreline at the campground.

ACCESS From the North Welcome Station, take Woodlands Trace south 9.0 miles to FR 133, Silver Trail Road. Turn left on Silver Trail Road and follow it 3.0 miles to FR 134. Turn right on FR 134 and follow it 4.1 miles to the dam. The boat ramps are on the far side of the dam.

■ GOLDEN POND VISITOR CENTER POND

STATE Kentucky   **LAKE ACREAGE** 2 acres   **OPEN** Year-round
USE Low to moderate   **SPECIAL REGULATIONS** None

THIS POND LIES between Woodlands Trace and Golden Pond Visitor Center. The attractive setting enhances the angling opportunities, especially for catfish. This pond is known for catfish. Families are often seen bank fishing here, usually with a picnic basket. Hardcore anglers head elsewhere.

ACCESS Golden Pond Visitor Center is centrally located at LBL. It can be reached from the east on I-24 at Exit 65 via US 68/KY 80, from the north on I-24 from Exit 31 via KY 453 South, from the west by KY 80, and from the south by US 79 and Woodlands Trace.

■ HEMATITE LAKE

STATE Kentucky   LAKE ACREAGE 90 acres
OPEN Boats, May 16–October 31; bank, March 16–October 31
USE High   SPECIAL REGULATIONS Electric motors only

HEMATITE LAKE IS an impoundment of Long Creek and is part of the Nature Station Environmental Education Area. It is popular with bank and boat anglers. The attractive lake is bordered by hills on both sides and a wetland in its upper section. A hiking trail extends around the lake. Come here if you want a scenic and rewarding fishing experience.

ACCESS From the entrance of Golden Pond Visitor Center, head north on Woodlands Trace 7 miles to Mulberry Flats Road, FR 135. Turn right on Mulberry Flats Road and follow it 4 miles to FR 134. Turn left on FR 134 and follow it 1 mile to Hematite Lake Picnic Area, on your left just before the Center Furnace ruins. The lake is at the upper end of the picnic area.

■ HONKER LAKE

STATE Kentucky   LAKE ACREAGE 190 acres
OPEN March 16–October 31; except two northwestern bays, May 16–October 31
USE Moderate   SPECIAL REGULATIONS No-wake lake

HONKER LAKE IS part of the Nature Station Environmental Education Area. It is one of two impoundments on Long Creek. Honker Lake is the lower impoundment and is separated from Lake Barkley only by a dam. Honker Lake has canoes for rent, in case anglers are without boats. A hiking trail encircles the lake, making bank fishing more viable. Boaters can put in their craft at the wildlife observation area near the beginning of the Long Creek Trail.

ACCESS From the entrance of Golden Pond Visitor Center, take Woodlands Trace 7 miles north to Mulberry Flat Road, FR 135. Turn right on Mulberry Flat Road and follow it 4 miles to FR 134. Turn left on FR 134 and follow it 1 mile to a right turn, passing the Long Creek Trailhead parking, just across from the Center Furnace ruins.

■ LONG CREEK

STATE Kentucky   **OPEN** Year-round   Use Low to moderate
SPECIAL REGULATIONS None

LONG CREEK OFFERS the only stream fishing at LBL. Nearly all surface streams in the recreation area dry up for part of the year. The fishable section of Long Creek remains flowing because Hematite Lake feeds it. Most folks bank fish Long Creek from the Hematite Lake Picnic Area. Others access the stream via the Long Creek Trail, which is just across the road from the picnic area. Anglers could use a kayak or canoe along this mile of creek.

ACCESS From the entrance of Golden Pond Visitor Center, head north on Woodlands Trace 7 miles to Mulberry Flats Road, FR 135. Turn right on Mulberry Flats Road and follow it 4 miles to FR 134. Turn left on FR 134 and follow it 1 mile to Hematite Lake Picnic Area, on your left just before Center Furnace ruins. Long Creek flows past the picnic area.

■ LONG CREEK POND

STATE Kentucky   **LAKE ACREAGE** 6 acres   **OPEN** May 16–October 31
USE Low   **SPECIAL REGULATIONS** None

THE LONG CREEK of this Long Creek Pond is different from the Long Creek near the Nature Station. Long Creek Pond is separated from Lake Barkley by US 68/KY 80, near Devils Elbow Lake Access Area. The road is the dam for this shallow lake surrounded by grassy fields. It looks attractive from the road, but the road noise can make it less than appealing as a fishing venue.

ACCESS From the entrance of Golden Pond Visitor Center, drive south a quarter mile to Golden Pond Road. Turn left on Golden Pond Road and follow it 0.3 mile to US 68/KY 80. Turn right, heading east, and follow US 68/KY 80 3.6 miles to FR 151. Turn left on FR 151 and Long Creek Pond is to your left.

Swim Beaches

WITH 300 MILES OF SHORELINE along Lake Barkley and Kentucky Lake and numerous lake access areas, swimming opportunities at Land Between The Lakes are limited only by your willingness to seek out a swimming hole or one of the designated swim beaches (the best choice, especially for families with kids). Two campgrounds have designated swim beaches, Piney and Hillman Ferry. However, these swim beaches are exclusively for the use of campers overnighting at the campground. Land Between The Lakes does have two other swim beaches available for day use, Energy Lake and Moss Creek Day-Use Area.

■ ENERGY LAKE

ENERGY LAKE SWIM BEACH is located inside Energy Lake Campground. Stop at the campground entrance station and pay the $2 per person fee (ages 4 and under, free) and continue a short distance to reach the beach.

The gravel road descends to a large grassy field beside the parking area. A playground and basketball court are near the field and the sandy swim beach is to the right with yellow floats delineating the swim area. A sloping hill broken with large shade trees overlooks the swim beach. Picnic tables and grills complement the hillside.

Placid waters

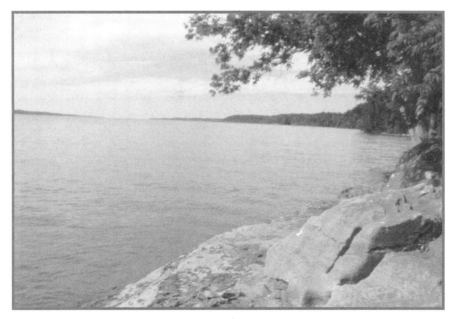

ACCESS From the North Welcome Station, take Woodlands Trace south 9.0 miles to FR 133, Silver Trail Road. Turn left on Silver Trail Road and follow it 3.0 miles to FR 134. Turn right on FR 134 and follow it 4.5 miles to the campground, on your right. The swim beach is inside the campground.

■ MOSS CREEK

MOSS CREEK DAY-USE AREA offers an attractive rock-and-gravel beach on the shores of Kentucky Lake. There is no user fee. Forest Road 106 takes you past homesites before dropping down a hill and reaching a lakeside flat. An ideal mix of trees, grass, and beach offers many combinations of sun and shade. The main beach is 60 yards long and offers expansive views up and down Kentucky Lake. The beach is backed by shade trees growing out of gravel. Behind the gravel are grassy areas, some shaded and some not. Amenities here include five picnic tables, five grills, and accessible vault toilets. The North–South Trail runs directly through the day-use area, offering hiking opportunities for those so inclined.

ACCESS From the North Welcome Station, head south on Woodlands Trace 0.6 mile to paved FR 106. Turn right on FR 106 and follow it 1.0 mile to reach the day-use area.

Lake Access Areas

GETTING ON THE WATER at LBL is relatively simple, with 15 lake access areas to facilitate your boat launch. The profiles in this section will help you determine which access area best meets your needs. Since the access point you choose will likely serve as a base camp for your LBL excursions, the profiles include information on facilities and activities available on-site and nearby. The "Nearest campground" field indicates the closest developed campground (see "Campgrounds," pages 160–176, for details on each). More basic camping is available at several access areas.

■ BOSWELL LANDING

LAKE Kentucky Lake   **NEAREST TOWN** Dover, TN   **ACCESS ROAD** Paved
NEAREST CAMPGROUND Piney   **OPEN** Year-round   **USE** Moderate to high
FACILITIES Courtesy dock, picnic tables, grills, tent pads, accessible vault toilets
ACTIVITIES Boating, fishing, hiking, camping

BOSWELL LANDING IS situated on a hilly point where Panther Bay meets Kentucky Lake. This promontory offers an outstanding view north, up Kentucky Lake as far as the sky allows, and eastward into Panther Bay and Dry Fork Bay. The launch ramp is protected by a small cove when the winds are high on Kentucky Lake. A courtesy dock extends into the water, making loading and unloading passengers easier.

A quality picnic/camping area with 23 level sites is situated on the hill; the Campbell Cemetery is located at the high point on the hill. Camping is allowed only after purchase of a backcountry camping permit. Boswell can get busy if nearby Piney Campground fills. The nearby picnic/campsites have concrete picnic tables and fire rings with built-in grills. Landscaping timbers keep the sites level and hold gravel for drainage around a tent or parking area of a camping rig. Most of the sites are too small for an RV, though a few of the sites closer to the lake will accommodate a big rig. A mix of exposed and shaded sites adds variety. Nine of the picnic/campsites are directly lakeside, with most of them overlooking the main body of Kentucky Lake, where you will see folks fishing off the bank. Water action has eroded some of the shoreline on Kentucky Lake and sent a few former sites into the water. Overall, Boswell is as nice as some fee campgrounds, but doesn't have potable water.

Hiking is an option here. The Fort Henry Trail System can be accessed at Boswell. At the upper end of the hill is Point 25 (numbered trail signs mark specific points in the trail system). From Point 25, the Boswell Trail leads 0.4 mile to the Picket Loop, so named for the Rebel posts guarding Fort Henry's perimeter. From Point 25, hikers can leave the landing and enjoy a 3-mile loop along the Panther Creek watershed. Get a trail map at the South Welcome Center before you hike.

You will pass a roadside marker noting the Civil War site of Fort Henry on the way in. It was at Fort Henry that the Confederacy set up a defense of the Tennessee River. However, on February 6, 1862, Union gunboats blasted the rebels into retreat toward Fort Donelson on the Cumberland River, setting up a second battle there.

ACCESS From the South Welcome Station, take FR 230, Fort Henry Road, 4.1 miles to FR 232. Turn right on FR 232 and follow it 0.1 mile to FR 233. Turn right on FR 233 and follow it 1.2 miles to dead-end at the landing.

■ DEMUMBERS BAY

LAKE Lake Barkley   **NEAREST TOWN** Grand Rivers, KY   **ACCESS ROAD** Paved
NEAREST CAMPGROUND Hillman Ferry   **OPEN** Year-round   **USE** Low
FACILITIES Picnic tables, accessible vault toilets   **ACTIVITIES** Boating, fishing, camping

DEMUMBERS BAY IS the sort of place that makes you wonder why it isn't more popular. It's nothing to jump up and down over, yet is quaint and secluded, especially in LBL's facility-concentrated far north end. But that may be why it is used so little—four other lake access areas are within 5 miles.

Be careful entering the lake access, as FR 108 heads directly into Lake Barkley. The actual access ramp shifts to the right before reaching the water. A low hill overlooks the upper end of Demumbers Bay. Five picnic tables are located on the perimeter of the gravel access. Most of them are shaded. Potential campsites beside the tables are small. Camping is allowed here with a backcountry permit. An old homesite 0.1 mile away from the lake also is used for camping. Big maples shade the homesite.

A large field lies to the right of the hill. From the ramp, you can look north into Lake Barkley. The ramp has a solid incline, but it is wide, making it usable by your average boater. Demumbers Bay offers decent shelter from the wind.

ACCESS From the North Welcome Station, take Woodlands Trace south 1.1 miles to paved FR 108. Turn left on FR 108 and follow it 2.0 miles to dead-end at the lake access. A short segment of the road is gravel as it crosses Willow Bay.

■ DEVILS ELBOW

LAKE Lake Barkley   **NEAREST TOWN** Canton, KY   **ACCESS ROAD** Gravel
NEAREST CAMPGROUND Energy Lake   **OPEN** Year-round   **USE** Low
FACILITIES Accessible vault toilets   **ACTIVITIES** Boating, fishing

DEVILS ELBOW IS named for a now-flooded bend in the Cumberland River. This landing has some big pluses and some big minuses. The actual boat ramp is first rate: A wide concrete ramp leads into a minibay off the Long Creek arm of Elbow Bay; it is shielded from wind by a small jetty. The minus: The area is just off US 68/KY 80, making for a noisy endeavor. If you can stand some car noise, this place will do.

Enter the landing. The Long Creek Cemetery stands on a hill to your left. A gravel road dives right down to a pond created by the elevated fill of the new highway to your right and the elevated fill of the old highway to your left. A little gravel beach fronts the pond. This pond is a fun place for kids to swim. Also, it is nice place to take a canoe or self-propelled boat and fish for bream. The main road keeps forward and goes over a hill where a home once stood. The sheltered boat ramp is on the far side of the hill. Old US 68/KY 80 leads right and crosses the Long Creek arm of Elbow Bay. Fishing is allowed from the rocky riprap on the bank of the old highway. Stores are conveniently located just across the Cumberland River in Canton.

ACCESS From the entrance of Golden Pond Visitor Center, drive south 0.25 mile to Golden Pond Road. Turn left on Golden Pond Road and follow it 0.3 mile to US 68/KY 80. Turn right, heading east, and follow US 68/KY 80 3.6 miles to the landing, on your right.

■ EDDYVILLE FERRY

LAKE Lake Barkley   **NEAREST TOWN** Grand Rivers, KY   **ACCESS ROAD** Paved
NEAREST CAMPGROUND Hillman Ferry   **OPEN** Year-round   **USE** Very low
FACILITIES None   **ACTIVITIES** Boating, fishing, camping

THE HISTORY OF THIS SPOT is evident after taking Old Ferry Road to Eddyville Ferry Lake Access. Before the Cumberland River was dammed, Between The Rivers residents took a ferry across the Cumberland to reach the east side of the river. Now, Old Ferry Road makes for a scenic drive through obviously once-settled land to end at a lonely boat launch.

Old Ferry Road leads directly into the boat ramp. A barricade has been constructed to keep unsuspecting motorists from launching themselves into the water prematurely. The continuation of Old Ferry Road is visible beyond the ramp. This raised roadbed helps keep the waves down at the launch, though Eddyville Ferry is in a small but wide cove.

A wide, paved rectangle makes for the only level spot at the lake access. The few campers who stay here "make do with what they got." Folks in rigs park their campers on the edge of the pavement. Tent campers throw up the canvas on the grassy edge, hoping they won't roll into the lake.

Old Eddyville was as awash in history as it is submerged today, beneath the waters of Lake Barkley. In 1801, former Vermont congressman Matthew Lyon led settlers from the Granite State to the banks of the Cumberland River, homesteading in what he called Eddy, later to become Eddyville. He and his son Chittenden established farms, stores, and even the first iron ore furnace in what is now LBL. Lyon County, which encompasses the northern third of LBL, was named for Lyon.

Eddyville Ferry sees very little traffic. It is the least-used lake access in the whole of LBL, so if you are looking for solitude, this is the lake access for you.

ACCESS From the North Welcome Station, take Woodlands Trace south 5.3 miles to paved FR 117, Old Ferry Road. Turn left on FR 117 and follow it 7.0 miles to a dead end at the landing.

■ ENERGY DAM

LAKE Energy Lake, Barkley   **NEAREST TOWN** Canton, KY   **ACCESS ROAD** Paved

NEAREST CAMPGROUND Energy Lake   **OPEN** Year-round   **USE** High

FACILITIES Accessible vault toilets   **ACTIVITIES** Boating, fishing, hiking

ENERGY DAM LAKE ACCESS AREA is part of the greater Energy Lake recreation complex. Energy Lake Campground is less than a mile away. However, Energy Dam receives heavy use from noncampers. Camping is not allowed at this spot, where two boat ramps serve two adjacent lakes, Energy Lake and Lake Barkley. Energy Lake is a no-wake lake.

Forest Road 134 crosses Energy Lake Dam. The rocky riprap on either side of the dam offers bank fishing spots. Bank fishing is very popular here. Be careful crossing the dam road, as vehicles are allowed to park on the Lake Barkley side of the dam.

An L-shaped courtesy dock and fishing pier extends into the water from the Lake Barkley boat ramp. The Lake Barkley boat ramp leads into Crooked Creek Bay and is less subject to Barkley's potential winds. Energy Lake, 370 acres, is less often a wind hazard. Both boat ramps are moderately sloped and easy to use.

You can combine fishing with self-propelled boating, as canoes are available for rent at Energy Lake Campground. If you want to hike, the Energy Lake Loop Trail starts at the campground entrance road. You can make a 2- or 4-mile loop. Get a trail map from the campground entrance station.

ACCESS From the North Welcome Station, take Woodlands Trace south 9.0 miles to FR 133, Silver Trail Road. Turn left on Silver Trail Road and follow it 3.0 miles to FR 134. Turn right on FR 134 and follow it 4.1 miles to the dam. The boat ramps are on the far side of the dam.

■ GINGER BAY

LAKE Kentucky Lake   **NEAREST TOWN** Dover, TN   **ACCESS ROAD** Gravel

NEAREST CAMPGROUND Piney   **OPEN** Year-round   **USE** Low to moderate

FACILITIES None   **ACTIVITIES** Boating, fishing, camping

THE LAST 2 MILES of this auto access are hilly and winding, so make sure you have the necessary power and traction to haul your boat. Once here, you will find Ginger Bay a primitive area. There are no facilities, except for the fairly steep concrete boat launch. It is officially designated a "low maintenance area," which means you pack out your trash. Bring everything you need too.

The landing is scenic. It sits on a point of land and overlooks the curving shoreline of Ginger Bay westward into Kentucky Lake. Rough campsites are located on a couple of spur roads just before reaching the boat launch. These areas overlook the bay but are nothing more than relatively level spots with primitive fire rings used by previous campers. A backcountry permit is required to camp here.

ACCESS From the South Welcome Station, take Woodlands Trace north 7.7 miles to FR 211, Ginger Bay Road. Turn left on paved FR 211 and follow it 1.6 miles. Keep forward as FR 211 becomes FR 206. Follow FR 206 1.7 more miles to gravel FR 212. Turn left on FR 212 and follow it 1.9 miles to the landing.

■ GRAYS LANDING

LAKE Kentucky Lake	**NEAREST TOWN** Dover, TN	**ACCESS ROAD** Gravel
NEAREST CAMPGROUND Piney	**OPEN** Year-round	**USE** Low to moderate
FACILITIES None	**ACTIVITIES** Boating, fishing, camping	

THIS LANDING IS on the site of a former homestead. Times have changed since the Gray clan lived here. The Tennessee River has been dammed and a massive concrete bridge spans what is now Kentucky Lake. The Gray Cemetery sits high on a hill overlooking the lake and bridge.

Grays Landing is primitive. It has no facilities. A short paved road leads to a small maze of rutted gravel roads leading down to and along the shore of Kentucky Lake. A concrete ramp lies close to the US 79 bridge. Although the landing is primitive, it is not rustic. The cars of US 79 roar by on the pavement and over the bridge. Despite the noise, primitive campsites are scattered in the area.

ACCESS From US 79 at the junction with Woodlands Trace, go south on US 79 8.8 miles to the landing, located on the right just before the bridge over Kentucky Lake.

■ KUTTAWA LANDING

LAKE Lake Barkley	**NEAREST TOWN** Grand Rivers, KY	**ACCESS ROAD** Gravel
NEAREST CAMPGROUND Hillman Ferry	**OPEN** Year-round	**USE** Very low
FACILITIES Picnic tables	**ACTIVITIES** Boating, fishing, camping	

KUTTAWA LANDING IS situated on a knoll overlooking a large bend in Lake Barkley. This bend was the last southward turn in what was the Cumberland River before it reverted north to reach the Ohio River. This nearly forgotten landing offers solitude for those wanting to be lakeside.

Arrive at the landing after questioning its existence on the drive in. A barricade keeps drivers from entering the river too suddenly. Come to a pretty, grassy knoll with a commanding view of Lake Barkley. The gravel road drops to the right and reaches a small but adequate boat ramp in a cove, sheltered from all but a north/northwest wind. Pass a small, flat area used by smaller rigs to camp. The road climbs the knoll and reaches three picnic/campsites beneath a couple of hackberry and maple trees. If you have a rig, it will be difficult to find a level locale for overnighting beside the picnic tables. A backcountry permit is required to camp at Kuttawa Landing. Picnickers will love their shaded vantage point beside the lake. Water sports are the name of the game here at the last gasp of the Cumberland River.

This Southern waterway is born on the Cumberland Plateau and in the mountains of eastern Kentucky and Tennessee. Its feeder streams are wild waterways of crashing rapids that cut through limestone bluffs of the plateau. Upon becoming the Cumberland, the river is dammed as Lake Cumberland, then once again freed. It enters Tennessee, where it is impounded first as Dale Hollow Lake, then Cordell Hull Lake, Old Hickory Lake, and finally Cheatham Lake. With one last push, it turns north and enters Kentucky as Lake Barkley, then flows into the Ohio River. However, since 1966, a canal that forms the northernmost border of LBL has joined the Cumberland and Tennessee Rivers.

ACCESS From the North Welcome Station, take Woodlands Trace south 7.0 miles to paved FR 117, Old Ferry Road. Turn left on FR 117 and follow it 6.4 miles to FR 126. Turn left on FR 126 and follow it 0.6 mile to FR 127. Veer right on FR 127 and follow it 1.2 miles to dead-end at the landing.

■ NEVILLE BAY

LAKE Lake Barkley	**NEAREST TOWN** Dover, TN	**ACCESS ROAD** Gravel
NEAREST CAMPGROUND Piney	**OPEN** Year-round	**USE** Low
FACILITIES Picnic tables, accessible vault toilets	**ACTIVITIES** Boating, fishing	

THIS LANDING IS located on attractive Neville Bay, an arm of Lake Barkley. Neville Creek and a small branch flowing out of Crutcher Hollow feed this bay. The landing is located on a gently sloping, mostly grassy hill. As you enter the access, a short gravel road leads right to two picnic tables and a vault toilet. These tables are partly shaded by cedar and hardwoods. This area commands a good view of the east–west running bay and into a bit of Lake Barkley, which is split by a long-running island. A hilly, wooded shoreline forms the backdrop for Neville Bay.

The main road descends to reach the concrete boat ramp. The mostly grassy hillside has three concrete picnic tables running perpendicular to the bay that enjoy afternoon shade from a line of trees. These three picnic tables have no immediate auto access—you have to carry your gear a bit to reach them.

Camping is allowed here with a backcountry camping permit. Activities are limited to boating and fishing. Neville Bay is a good jumping-off point for a scenic forest drive on gravel FR 214 beyond the part that you drove to get here. See South Loop Forest Drive (see "Scenic Drives," pages 153–154). Several homesites lie along the road. In places, the road bisects steep ravines cut with streams shaded in beech trees. Return to Woodlands Trace via FR 204.

ACCESS   From the South Welcome Station, take Woodlands Trace north 6.1 miles to FR 214, Neville Bay Road. Turn right on FR 214 and follow it 1.5 miles to the landing, on your right.

■ NICKELL BRANCH

LAKE Lake Barkley   **NEAREST TOWN** Grand Rivers, KY   **ACCESS ROAD** Gravel
NEAREST CAMPGROUND Hillman Ferry   **OPEN** Year-round   **USE** Moderate
FACILITIES Picnic tables, grills, courtesy dock, accessible vault toilets
ACTIVITIES Boating, fishing, mountain biking, hiking, camping

NICKELL BRANCH IS a busier boat ramp. For travelers entering LBL from the north, it is the first boat ramp encountered. In summer, boaters from nearby Paducah use Nickell Branch to access Lake Barkley. The canal connecting Lake Barkley to Kentucky Lake is close to Nickell Branch, so boaters can motor just a short distance to also reach Kentucky Lake.

After leaving Woodlands Trace, reach a grassy hill with a vista of Lake Barkley. Descend along a gravel loop and reach the ramp, entering the lake along the Nickell Branch arm of Lake Barkley. A bad wind from the northeast might affect launching, but the moderate slope makes for easy entry and exit in the water.

Near the boat ramp, two nice picnic/campsites are set directly lakeside beneath tree cover. More sites are on a bluff overlooking the lake and Barkley Dam. These sites are shaded. The main loop road curves up a hill past several small sites that are shaded by hackberry trees with a grassy understory. Most of the sites are not level and don't have a place to pull up your rig or pitch your tent. These sites are better suited for picnicking. Backcountry permits are required to camp here. An accessible vault toilet building serves the area.

Although this lake access receives a lot of aquatic use, boaters are not the only ones to stay here. Mountain bikers will use Nickell Branch as a jumping-off point, since the Canal Loop Trail passes through here at the top of the hill. This trail system allows for loop rides and hikes ranging from 1.5 miles to 14 miles in length. Kentucky Lake Drive makes for a short, scenic auto tour. The North Welcome Station is nearby for information. The town of Grand Rivers is just north of here for quick supply runs.

ACCESS From the North Welcome Station, take Woodlands Trace north 1.0 mile to FR 102. Turn right on FR 102 and follow it 0.9 mile to dead-end at the landing.

■ PISGAH POINT

LAKE Kentucky Lake   **NEAREST TOWN** Grand Rivers, KY   **ACCESS ROAD** Gravel
NEAREST CAMPGROUND Hillman Ferry   **OPEN** Year-round   **USE** Low
FACILITIES Picnic tables, courtesy dock, accessible vault toilets
ACTIVITIES Boating, fishing, hiking, mountain biking, camping

PISGAH POINT HAS decent natural attributes—it's just a little worn around the edges. The gravel access road leads along a ridge, passing the fenced Lee Cemetery, and descends to the landing, which looks south over the bay. An inlet across the bay opens to Kentucky Lake beyond. Mostly grass and some trees surround the landing, which has seen better days. A few level spots and picnic tables are spread around Pisgah Point. The boat ramp is adequate and should accommodate most watercraft. Primitive spur roads lead to rough lakeside campsites up Pisgah Bay. Away from the lake, other spur roads lead to other rough campsites. A backcountry permit is required to camp here. Birmingham Ferry Campground is visible across the water.

Anglers use this camp for bank and boat fishing. Hikers and mountain bikers should note the North–South Trail crosses FR 111 just steps from the lake access. Trail travelers can check out Nightriders Spring and its trail shelter just north of Pisgah Point or keep north and ride the roads upon reaching Hillman Ferry Campground. Southbounders can trek the length of Pisgah Bay, circling around Pisgah

Creek to reach Old Ferry Road, which leads around to the far side of Pisgah Bay. Lee Cemetery, atop Pisgah Point, attests to the historical element of LBL. Please honor the intent of the fence here.

ACCESS   From the North Welcome Station, take Woodlands Trace south 3.1 miles to paved FR 111. Turn right on FR 111, staying left at 0.1 mile as it turns to gravel. Follow it 1.8 miles to end at the landing.

■ REDD HOLLOW

LAKE Kentucky Lake   **NEAREST TOWN** Aurora, KY   **ACCESS ROAD** Gravel
NEAREST CAMPGROUND Wranglers   **OPEN** Year-round   **USE** Low
FACILITIES Picnic tables, grills, tent pads, accessible vault toilets
ACTIVITIES Boating, fishing, hiking, camping

REDD HOLLOW IS one of the more developed lake access areas. It offers over 30 picnic/campsites in addition to a standard boat ramp. While driving down Redd Hollow to the landing, imagine it as an 1800s tannery area. Here, hides from the area's abundant animals were processed. Tannin was obtained from the trees of Redd

Camping at Redd Hollow

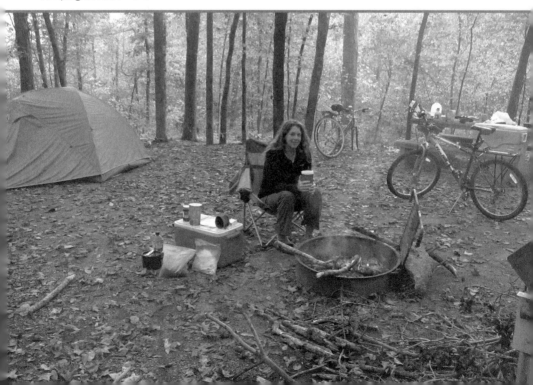

Hollow and the hides were soaked in water from springs along this stream. A lot of hard human labor went into scraping the fur off the hides. When finished, the hides were sold locally or shipped out on the nearby Tennessee River.

Nowadays, the Tennessee River at this point is dammed as Kentucky Lake. The bay of Redd Hollow is short, allowing wide views into the lake, especially from the many stunning picnic/campsites here. The first set of sites is strung along the lower end of the hollow, deep in the shade. Farther down, many sites overlook the bay and, southward, the lake, offering a mixture of sun and shade. A gravel loop curves over a hill and offers sites on high land that look down on the lake to the west and north. Of special note is site 31. It stands alone at the highest point of the hill and commands a view of the lake and Redd Hollow.

Camping is allowed here after purchase of a backcountry camping permit. And you will want to do that after seeing the abundance of attractive sites. However, an accessible vault toilet building is your only amenity. The sites do have concrete picnic tables, fire grates, and level tent pads. Bring your own water.

Boating and fishing are natural pursuits. Hikers do have the option of picking up the Mountain Laurel Spring Spur Trail located a mile up Redd Hollow toward Woodlands Trace. The trail leads right a short distance to Mountain Laurel Spring and left 0.8 mile to the North–South Trail. Along the way to the North–South Trail, the spur trail passes one of the largest stands of mountain laurel in LBL. Mountain laurel, which blooms a profusion of pinkish-white blooms in late April and early May, is becoming rare in these parts.

ACCESS From the entrance of the Golden Pond Visitor Center, take Woodlands Trace south 4.7 miles to FR 171. Turn right on FR 171 and follow it 1.7 miles to a dead end at the landing.

■ SUGAR BAY

LAKE Kentucky Lake   NEAREST TOWN Aurora, KY   ACCESS ROAD Gravel
NEAREST CAMPGROUND Energy Lake   OPEN Year-round   USE Low to moderate
FACILITIES Picnic tables, grills, accessible vault toilets
ACTIVITIES Boating, fishing, hiking, mountain biking, camping

SUGAR BAY LAKE Access is actually set in the South Fork Sugar Creek arm of Sugar Bay. This makes for a tight, close-knit setting among the steep hills and carved hollows in this little-visited yet quality locale. The road leading into this lake access is pretty steep and winding in places, discouraging those with larger boats. But once here, you can fish this bay, have a hilltop picnic, or camp. A backcountry permit is required for overnight use of Sugar Bay.

Two picnic/campsites are in a lone hollow away from the lake as soon as you arrive. The gravel road splits at the hollow. One gravel road leads uphill to nine sites atop a knob overlooking the water on either side. The sites are spread far apart, allowing for privacy beneath the forest. Dropping back down to the lake, a few sites are located in the upper end of the bay in bottomland. I wouldn't want to be camped there when a big rain hits. A road curves around to the boat launch. The boat ramp itself is on a smaller arm of the South Fork Sugar Creek arm. It has a fine ramp suitable for smaller boats that could make it in here. Boater parking sites are limited.

Fishing and boating are the primary activities here, but hiking and mountain biking are options. The North–South Trail passes just a stone's throw from the lake access entrance. Walk a little bit up Ironton Road from Sugar Bay and you will reach the white-blazed path. To your right, the North–South Trail leaves south to Higgins Bay. To your left, the trail heads north to the Sugar Jack Spring Spur Trail. Located on North Fork Sugar Creek, the spring water was once used for making moonshine.

ACCESS From the entrance of Golden Pond Visitor Center, take Woodlands Trace north 5.7 miles to FR 140, Ironton Road. Turn left on FR 140 and follow it 2.1 miles to dead-end at Sugar Bay.

■ TAYLOR BAY

LAKE Lake Barkley   **NEAREST TOWN** Canton, KY   **ACCESS ROAD** Paved
NEAREST CAMPGROUND Energy Lake   **OPEN** Year-round   **USE** Low to moderate
FACILITIES Picnic tables, grills, accessible vault toilets, courtesy dock
ACTIVITIES Boating, fishing, camping

TAYLOR BAY IS an attractive spot—it looks almost as if it should be a fee campground. The 31 picnic/campsites are well kept, and the ramp is in good condition. But it is classified as a lake access area and no fees are charged, whether you are using it for launching your boat or day use. A backcountry camping permit is required for overnight use of Taylor Bay.

Follow the paved road to the lake access overlooking intimate Taylor Bay, which is fed by Taylor Creek. A side road leads right along an oak ridge. Seventeen picnic/campsites are stretched along the road. They are well shaded and a little close together. However, if you choose this area, you will likely have privacy—the sites don't ever fully fill here. Actually, this oak ridge is the place to go if you want solitude at Taylor Bay.

The main gravel loop descends to Taylor Bay. Four larger picnic/campsites are located near the wide, easy boat ramp. A courtesy dock floats next to the ramp. The little bay protects boats from the wind. Some of the most coveted sites are stretched out on the lakeside part of the loop. The loop turns away from Lake Barkley onto a hill. A few more sites are located in the center of the loop, which is mostly open, save for a large aspen tree in the center.

Taylor Bay is an angler's camp. For those inclined otherwise, the nearby Energy Lake area offers hiking trails, as does the Nature Station. The Nature Station is a comprehensive environmental education center on Honker and Hematite Lakes, where you can see animals up close, enjoy waterside hikes, and learn about the animals and plants of LBL. Canoes may be rented too. The Nature Station is open from March through November.

ACCESS From the entrance of Golden Pond Visitor Center, take Woodlands Trace north 7.0 miles to paved FR 135, Mulberry Flats Road. Turn right on FR 135 and follow it 4.8 miles to FR 136. Turn right on FR 136 and follow it 0.4 mile to a dead end at Taylor Bay.

■ TWIN LAKES

LAKE Kentucky Lake   **NEAREST TOWN** Grand Rivers, KY   **ACCESS ROAD** Gravel
NEAREST CAMPGROUND Hillman Ferry   **OPEN** Year-round   **USE** Low
FACILITIES Picnic tables, vault toilets
ACTIVITIES Boating, fishing, mountain biking, hiking, camping

TWIN LAKES OUGHT to be called "Twin Coves." The lake access area is broken into two parts, each part on small coves of Kentucky Lake. A low ridge separates the two coves, the bigger of which lies beside the picnic/camp area. Drop into the first cove from Woodlands Trace. A road leads right to a series of picnic/campsites. The first section forms a loop with several picnic tables, some with grills, around the loop. Some sites open to the sun are in the middle of the loop. Continue along the edge of the cove to reach some lakeside sites. Just a bit down are hilltop sites looking southwest over Kentucky Lake. These are the best sites. A discriminating picnicker or camper will find a suitable spot. Camping is allowed with a backcountry permit. Vault toilets are stationed here and at the boat launch.

Continue beyond the picnic/camp area on gravel FR 105. It leads 0.6 mile to the actual ramp area, which has a rougher edge than the picnic/camp area. A couple of picnic tables are here too. Some primitive campsites connected by mud roads lie on the lake. The ramp is protected by a small cove and will serve your average LBL boater. Parking is limited in the ramp area, which has seen better days.

Mountain bikers and hikers take note that the North–South Trail passes directly through the boat launch area and near the picnic/camp area. An easy loop is made using the North–South Trail and FR 105. The North–South Trail also connects to the Moss Creek Day-Use Area with its gravel beach. On the way in, you crossed the North End Hike/Bike Trail. It provides more loop possibilities. Consult the LBL trail map, available at the North Welcome Station.

ACCESS From the North Welcome Station, take Woodlands Trace south 0.4 mile to paved FR 104. Turn right on FR 104 and follow it 0.3 mile to reach the picnic/camp area. The boat ramp is 0.6 mile beyond on gravel FR 105.

PART THREE

The Trails

How to Use the Trail Information

AT THE TOP OF EACH HIKE is an information box that allows the hiker quick access to pertinent information: trail type, difficulty, length, use, condition, highlights, and trail connections. Below is an example of a box included with a hike:

■ HEMATITE TRAIL

TYPE Foot only   **DIFFICULTY** Easy   **LENGTH** 2.2 miles
USE Moderate to heavy   **CONDITION** Good
HIGHLIGHTS Wildlife viewing, boardwalk, photo blind, big trees
CONNECTIONS Center Furnace Trail, Long Creek Trail

FROM THE INFORMATION BOX, the reader can see that the trail is for foot travel only. It could be any combination of foot, horse, or bicycle. The Hematite Trail is rated easy, which means it is level and the footing is good. "Difficulty" can be rated easy, moderate, or difficult. The Hematite Trail is 2.3 miles in length and moderately used. "Trail use," defined as how frequent the path is traveled, can be low, moderate, or high. "Condition" indicates the quality and maintenance of the trail bed. A rough or overgrown trail is considered in poor condition. "Highlights" naturally vary from trail to trail, but may include sights or activities. "Connections" tell readers what other trails intersect the trail described. The Hematite Trail connects to the Center Furnace Trail and the Long Creek Trail. This way you can look up these other trails for potential loops or extended one-way trips. The primary highlight of this trail is wildlife viewing.

Following each box is a running narrative of the hike. A detailed account follows, where trail junctions, stream crossings, and trailside features are noted along with their distance from the trailhead. This helps keep you apprised of your whereabouts as well as makes sure you don't miss those features noted. At the end of each narrative are detailed directions to reach the trailhead.

The trail profiles have been divided into groups according to the areas they cover and, to some extent, type. Within the groups, profiles appear alphabetically. The Canal

Loop Trails section covers the hiking and biking trails at the recreation area's north end. The Energy Lake Trails section covers the trails near Energy Lake Campground. The Fort Donelson Trails section covers the paths at the Civil War Battlefield just south of LBL near Dover, Tennessee. The Fort Henry Trails section covers the network of paths in LBL's south end. The Nature Station Trails section covers the Environmental Education Area paths. The North–South Trail is LBL's premier long-distance path. It extends the length of the recreation area from south to north. The North–South Spur Trails are included to avail loops and side trips from the North–South Trail. The Wranglers Trails are a network of bridle paths for use by equestrians in north-central LBL.

Within each section is a description of every marked and maintained trail within that area. That way, you can flip through the trails of each section and see which trails appeal to you. And if you don't feel like developing a trip of your own, following the trail descriptions is a section of suggested loop hikes for hikers and/or bikers covering the national recreation area. Flip through the book and find the trails most appealing to you, then get out there and explore LBL!

Canal Loop Trails

THE CANAL LOOP TRAILS are in LBL's North End. These paths are very popular with mountain bikers. Hikers are well represented too. The primary path, the Canal Loop Trail, makes an 11-mile circuit around the northernmost portion of the LBL peninsula. Other trails cut across the Canal Loop Trail, making possible loops from just over a mile to the full 14 miles. The North Paved Trail connects the North Welcome Station to the access road reaching Hillman Ferry Campground. The North–South Trail also ties into the Canal Loop Trails, adding more trail trekking possibilities. Trail maps are available at the North Welcome Station and online.

■ CANAL LOOP TRAIL

TYPE Foot and bicycle   **DIFFICULTY** Moderate to difficult   **LENGTH** 10.8 miles
USE Heavy   **CONDITION** Mostly good
HIGHLIGHTS Views of Lake Barkley and Kentucky Lake, loop possibilities
CONNECTIONS North–South Trail, Trail Connector A, Trail Connector B, Trail Connector C, Trail Connector D, North Paved Trail

THE CANAL LOOP TRAIL is the premier mountain biking trail at Land Between The Lakes. It circles the northernmost portion of the LBL peninsula, exploring nearly

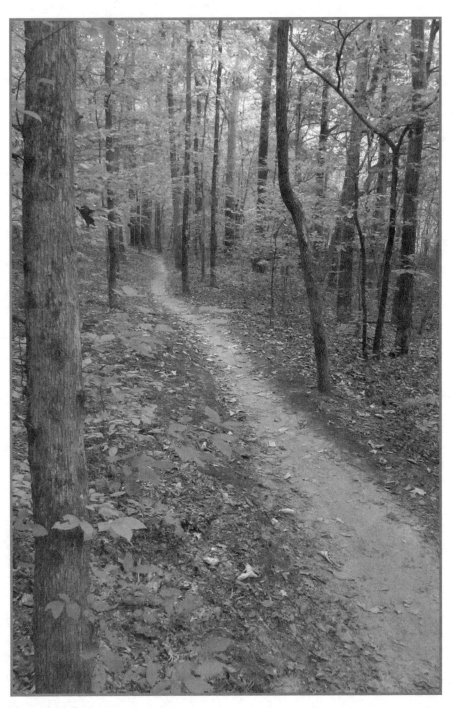

Canal Loop Trail

every environment the recreation area offers. The hills of the Canal Loop Trail challenge trail trekkers, yet offer great lake views of both Lake Barkley and Kentucky Lake. The Lake Barkley side of the loop is generally less hilly. Some rugged and regular ups and downs characterize the last portion of the path. Four connector trails make loop trips viable and allow spontaneous altering of loop lengths. You are likely to see the big barges that ply these waterways on the shoreline portions of these trails.

The Canal Loop Trail starts at the North Welcome Station. The trail begins beside a cypress tree in the median beside Woodlands Trace. Leave the North Welcome Station and cross Woodlands Trace. The Canal Loop Trail immediately spans a streambed on a wooden bridge. Here, a blue-blazed spur trail leads right a short distance south to Forest Road 302.

The blue-blazed Canal Loop Trail keeps forward, topping a low hill. The singletrack path descends to Nickell Branch in a heavily wooded hollow. Level out near Lake Barkley at 0.6 mile. Turn uphill, away from Nickell Branch, and pass a few concrete blockhouses. Use your imagination to guess their former use.

Pass under a power line at mile 1.1. Don't cross the adjoining forest road. Instead, keep right and reenter woods, back on singletrack. Descend to a rough boat launch and begin cruising alongside the Nickell Creek embayment. Islands of Lake Barkley are visible in the distance. Span a wooden bridge, then turn uphill, only to drop to the next embayment. Nickell Branch Lake Access is visible across the water. Curve around the feeder streams of this embayment, spanning a wooden bridge to reach a trail junction at mile 2.1. Here, Trail Connector C leaves left 0.7 mile to bisect the Canal Loop Trail in the Tennessee River watershed.

The Canal Loop Trail leaves right, beyond the bridge, to cross small feeder branches and come back alongside Lake Barkley. Suddenly, curve away from the water and snake steeply uphill to meet FR 102 at mile 2.8. Nickell Branch Lake Access is just down the hill to the right on FR 102. The Canal Loop Trail keeps forward, passing under a small power line twice to soon reach the lakeshore. Begin a pattern of curving away from the lake and returning to the shore. Reach a grassy area on a bluff at mile 3.4. This spot offers a great vista of Barkley Dam and the entrance to the canal connecting Lakes Barkley and Kentucky.

Beyond the vista, pass around a couple of smaller embayments before turning away from Lake Barkley for good. Keep on the edge of forest with a large field to the trail's right. The field gives way and the Canal Loop Trail passes under a power line. Cross a pair of bridges over stream branches in a flat. Reach a trail junction at mile 4.9. Trail Connector B leaves left 0.5 mile to shortcut the Canal Loop Trail.

The Canal Loop Trail turns away from a field to top a low hill. It then comes very near Woodlands Trace and reaches Trail Connector A at mile 5.4. Here, Trail Connector A leaves left 0.5 mile to reach the west side of the Canal Loop Trail. Keep forward past Connector A, coming alongside the Lake Barkley–Kentucky Lake Canal at mile 5.6. Interestingly, the current of the canal depends on which river watershed, the Tennessee or Cumberland, has received more rainfall lately.

The Canal Loop Trail keeps on a high bluff overlooking the canal, before curving around a small creek bed, then heads under Woodlands Trace at mile 5.8. Keep forward, gaining more canal and lake views to emerge onto Kentucky Lake Scenic Drive. Cross paved Kentucky Lake Scenic Drive. Keep forward into woods and reach a short spur trail, which leaves right, to trail access parking off Kentucky Lake Scenic Drive at mile 6.0. Leave the trailhead and keep a field to your right. Curve around a hollow then reach Trail Connector A at 6.4 miles. Trail Connector A leaves left 0.5 mile to the east side of Canal Loop Trail and forms the shortest loop in the trail system.

The Canal Loop Trail keeps forward alongside a field, which soon gives way to woods. Span a streambed on a wooden bridge and climb to reach a bluff at 6.8 miles. Begin heading inland on a hilltop and reach Trail Connector B at 7.1 miles. Trail Connector B leaves left 0.5 mile toward Lake Barkley. Keep forward on the blue-blazed path along a hickory-oak ridge. Begin working downhill into and down a narrow hollow. Crisscross a streambed to reach paved Kentucky Lake Scenic Drive. Cross the scenic drive and enter a potentially wet flat. Span back-to-back bridges to reach a trail junction at 7.8 miles. Trail Connector C leaves left here for 0.7 mile to reach the east side of the Canal Loop Trail near Nickell Branch Lake Access.

Turn back down toward Kentucky Lake, only to turn away and ascend a hollow onto a ridgeline. The Canal Loop Trail curves parallel to the shoreline on a tall bluff above a stream. Dip into a hollow where big vines snake around the trees. Climb steeply from the hollow via switchbacks back onto the bluff. The singletrack path opens to the tail end of FR 103. Keep along the bluff to soon turn away from the rough road back onto singletrack trail at mile 8.7. Dramatic vistas open among the hardwoods. This view once looked over some of Kentucky's most fertile farmland. Ironically, it was flooded to save lands elsewhere from flooding.

Switchback to a flat off the bluff. A campsite lies beside Kentucky Lake. The Canal Loop Trail makes a challenging ascent out of the flat to a rocky ridgeline. Grab a quick view before the trail drops to the next hollow south, only to climb again. The trail levels off and reaches a trail junction at mile 9.7. Here, Trail Connector D leaves left 0.8 mile to reach the North Welcome Station.

Keep forward on the Canal Loop Trail, dipping toward Kentucky Lake. Come alongside a bluff with a lake view before turning away from the lake and dropping into a hollow. Bisect a small flat before working back up to a rocky point with good views of the lake. Turn up a gravel ridgeline with an embayment to your right. The Twin Lakes Lake Access is visible across the embayment.

Drift to a hollow at the head of the embayment and cross a small branch on a wooden bridge at 10.6 miles. Intersect the North–South Trail. It has come nearly 60 miles from the South Welcome Station. The Canal Loop Trail turns left and joins the North–South Trail for the last 0.2 mile to North Welcome Station. The two trails pass through a potentially wet area. Reach an old blacktop road within sight of the North Welcome Station. Stay right and finally turn left on the North End Hike/Bike Trail to end the loop.

ACCESS This trail starts at the North Welcome Station. From Exit 31 on I-24 near Lake City, head south on KY 453 for 7 miles. (KY 453 becomes Woodlands Trace once it enters Land Between The Lakes National Recreation Area.)

■ NORTH PAVED TRAIL

TYPE Foot and bicycle   **DIFFICULTY** Easy   **LENGTH** 1.5 miles
USE Heavy   **CONDITION** Good
HIGHLIGHTS Good family trail, loop potential with North–South Trail
CONNECTIONS North–South Trail, Canal Loop Trail, Trail Connector D

THE NORTH PAVED TRAIL is the first experience for many LBL visitors. Families on bikes and on foot sample the recreation area on this path, which leaves the North Welcome Station and heads south through woods and fields to end at Forest Road 110, the access road for Hillman Ferry Campground. Campers at Hillman Ferry can use the hike/bike trail to access the Canal Loop Trails.

Start the paved trail near the flagpole at the North Welcome Station. Head south to enter woodland, after the combined North–South Trail and the Canal Loop Trail leave right on a paved road circling around the North Welcome Station picnic area. At 0.2 mile, cross paved FR 104. Shortly, come alongside Woodlands Trace to bisect paved FR 106 at 0.7 mile. Look right, just after the road crossing, for a beaver dam. Beavers have historically dammed the waters here.

Climb away from the beaver dam to pass by the Nickell Cemetery. Over 200 graveyards have been preserved at LBL, interring the former residents of this land. The stones range from unidentifiable fieldstones to two-tiered monuments. Cross FR 107 at mile 1.1. The North Paved Trail descends on a wider path flanked with locust trees, then leaves right, back into thick woods. Snake around a small streamshed before dipping to reach FR 110 at 1.5 miles. From here, it is right on FR 110 just a short distance to the North–South Trail, which also crosses FR 110, and just a bit farther to the Hillman Ferry Campground entrance. Trail users can backtrack on the hike/bike trail, or take the North–South Trail 3.8 miles back to the North Welcome Station.

ACCESS This trail starts at the North Welcome Station. From Exit 31 on I-24 near Lake City, head south on KY 453 for 7 miles. (KY 453 becomes Woodlands Trace once it enters Land Between The Lakes National Recreation Area.) It leaves south from the welcome station flagpole.

■ TRAIL CONNECTOR A

TYPE Foot and bicycle   **DIFFICULTY** Easy   **LENGTH** 0.5 mile
USE Moderate to heavy   **CONDITION** Good
HIGHLIGHTS Makes shortest loop in Canal Loop Trail System
CONNECTIONS Canal Loop Trail

THIS SHORT CONNECTOR PATH avails a loop of 1.4 miles from the Kentucky Lake Scenic Drive trailhead. Begin Trail Connector A on the Canal Loop Trail 0.3 mile south of the Kentucky Lake Scenic Drive trailhead. Head up along a washed-out streambed to level out at an old homesite—see the large trees amid a young forest. Also, look for the standing and fallen dead trunks of locust trees amid a taller forest of hackberry and other more shade-tolerant species. The locust invaded the old fields around the homesite, providing shade so the hackberry and other trees could grow.

Bisect a closed but paved road and dip to a power line. Cross Woodlands Trace to reenter woodland. Gently descend to meet the Canal Loop Trail. From here, it is 0.6 mile to the Kentucky Lake Scenic Drive trailhead.

ACCESS This is an interior trail. It can be reached by heading 0.3 mile south on the Canal Loop Trail from the Kentucky Lake Scenic Drive trailhead, which is a mile north of the North Welcome Station on Woodlands Trace. Once you reach Kentucky Lake Scenic Drive, turn left and follow it for a short distance to a gravel parking area on your left.

■ TRAIL CONNECTOR B

TYPE Foot and bicycle   **DIFFICULTY** Easy   **LENGTH** 0.5 mile
USE Moderate   **CONDITION** Good

HIGHLIGHTS Adds loop possibilities for Canal Loop Trails
CONNECTIONS Canal Loop Trail

TRAIL CONNECTOR B makes loops possible from the north and south. It begins in a flat along a feeder branch of the Cumberland River and climbs a bit over to the Tennessee River watershed and the western half of the Canal Loop Trail. Begin Trail Connector B at mile 4.9 of the Canal Loop Trail. The yellow-blazed path leaves a flat and heads uphill to reach Woodlands Trace at 0.1 mile. Cross Woodlands Trace. A decrepit paved road leaves right. Trail Connector B keeps forward past a telephone pole to dip into a clearing beneath a power line. The singletrack path crosses a streambed then climbs along a fence line through a young forest.

Reach a gravel road leading to a microwave tower. Follow the road left a short distance, then look for the yellow blazes leading right, away from the road and into the woods. Pass through a small clearing, then intersect the Canal Loop Trail. Here, the Canal Loop Trail leads right 1.1 miles back to the Kentucky Lake Scenic Drive trailhead.

ACCESS Trail Connector B is an interior trail. The east end starts at mile 4.9 along the Canal Loop Trail and the west end starts at mile 7.8 of the Canal Loop Trail.

■ TRAIL CONNECTOR C

TYPE Foot and bicycle   **DIFFICULTY** Easy   **LENGTH** 0.7 mile
USE Moderate to heavy   **CONDITION** Good
HIGHLIGHTS Adds loop possibilities to Canal Loop Trail
CONNECTIONS Canal Loop Trail

TRAIL CONNECTOR C is used to shortcut the Canal Loop Trail. Campers at Nickell Branch Lake Access use it since the trail's east end is very near them. Trail Connector C heads southwest up an old roadbed from mile 2.1 of the Canal Loop Trail, just after the bridge over a feeder stream near the lake access.

Leave the streamside flat and soon pass under a power line. Keep up the feeder branch valley, passing beside overturned concrete steps from a nearby homesite. Reach Woodlands Trace at 0.3 mile. Cross the paved road and reenter woods, running alongside Kentucky Lake Drive to your right. The trail becomes rooty as it works along a hillside. Kentucky Lake Drive turns away. Trail Connector C passes under a power line and over a wooden bridge just before intersecting the Canal Loop Trail at 7.8 miles.

ACCESS This is an interior trail. The east end of this trail starts at mile 2.1 on the Canal Loop Trail, which it reintersects at mile 7.8.

■ TRAIL CONNECTOR D

TYPE Foot and bicycle   **DIFFICULTY** Easy   **LENGTH** 0.8 mile

USE Heavy   **CONDITION** Good

HIGHLIGHTS Connects to trails directly from North Welcome Station

CONNECTIONS Canal Loop Trail, North–South Trail, North Paved Trail

THIS CONNECTOR TRAIL is popular because it starts at the North Welcome Station. Bikers and hikers can use it, a portion of the Canal Loop Trail, and the North–South Trail to make a good break-in circuit for LBL visitors. The trail begins at the trail signboard on the west side of the North Welcome Station parking area. Look for a sign labeled with the letter "D." Head across a low swale of grass to a sign beside a wooden bridge. Another white plastic sign notes this as Trail Connector D. Walk down the grassy area to reach the bridge. Cross the bridge and enter a hickory-oak woodland. The yellow-blazed path passes a rusty metal tank to the left of the trail. Trail Connector D makes several switchbacks up a hill before briefly dipping over a sunken roadbed. Climb a bit, then pass under a power line at 0.3 mile. The trail levels off on a ridgeline, making easy tracks to meet the Canal Loop Trail at 0.8 mile. The Canal Loop Trail leaves left 0.8 mile to join the North–South Trail and return to the North Welcome Station.

ACCESS This trail starts at the North Welcome Station. From Exit 31 on I-24 near Lake City, head south on KY 453 for 7.0 miles. (KY 453 becomes Woodlands Trace once it enters Land Between The Lakes National Recreation Area.)

Hillman Heritage Trail

HILLMAN HERITAGE TRAIL, a network of interconnected loops open to hikers and bicyclers, is a federally designated national recreation trail adjacent to Hillman Ferry Campground that presents a chance to hike or bike your way through a historic parcel of LBL, mixed in with the natural beauty for which the area is known. The 5.5-mile trail complex mostly follows old roads used by former residents of LBL, mixed in with some newly created pathways. The trails explore the greater Star Lime Works area. The lime business provided jobs for the residents, many of whom lived nearby. Historical interpretive information complements the trail system. Be apprised that although trails are open to bicyclers, short grades can be steep, and a little mountain biking skill will help you navigate sharp turns, occasional inclines, and irregular terrain. Four loops comprise the bulk of the trail mileage. The Bohannon Loop is the longest at 2.1 miles and provides linkage to all the other circuits. The Vogle Loop heads out a peninsula, passing

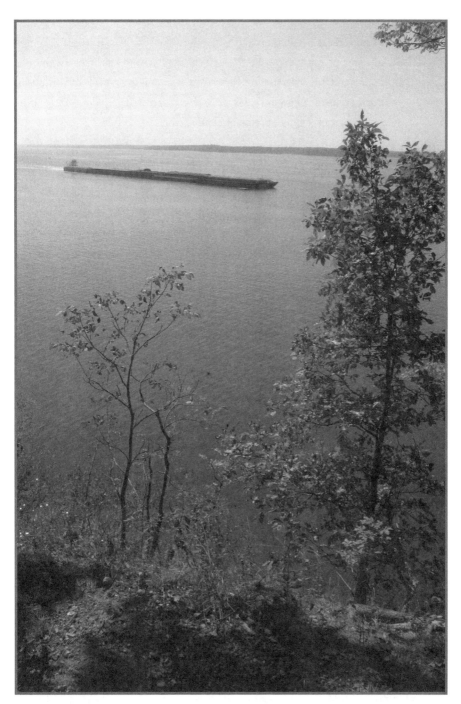

Vista on James Nickell Loop

a partly submerged quarry, homesites, a lake vista, a beach, and a second quarry. The Brown Spring Loop circles a highland ridge while the James Nickell Loop is highlighted with a fantastic vista of Kentucky Lake. Though the trail system starts inside Hillman Ferry Campground and is heavily used by campers, the path is open to all and includes a parking area outside the campground gates. However, please register your vehicle at the Hillman Ferry Campground gatehouse before embarking.

■ HILLMAN HERITAGE TRAIL: Bohannon Loop

TYPE Bicycle and foot   **DIFFICULTY** Moderate   **LENGTH** 2.1 miles
USE High   **CONDITION** Good, some rough spots
HIGHLIGHTS Bohannon Cemetery, homesites
CONNECTIONS Pinnegar Trail, Roy Young Trail, Vogle Loop, Connectors

THE BOHANNON LOOP is most often accessed via the main trailhead, after climbing a quarter mile from the Hillman Ferry gatehouse. Heading counterclockwise, the Bohannon Loop, shaded by towering hardwoods and occasional cedars, first passes a connector leaving left to the campground, then a spur leads right to the Bohannon Cemetery. Here, a fence encircles a few stone graves. Next, a connector leaves left, also heading to the campground. Then, the Pinnegar Trail leaves right 0.3 mile to shortcut the Bohannon Loop and also meet the short 0.1-mile Roy Young Trail. The Bohannon Loop then descends a rutted old road, passing a smokehouse site and old cellar to reach a trail intersection at 0.7 mile. Here, the Vogle Loop leaves left to make its mile-long circuit. The Bohannon Loop turns right on irregular trail, up and down to pass the Roy Young Trail at 1.1 miles. It then climbs a hill to meet the other end of the Pinnegar Trail at 1.3 miles. The Bohannon Loop undulates north to find a connector leaving left at 1.9 miles. The connector heads over a wide level ridge to the Brown Spring Loop. However, the Bohannon Loop leaves right and rolls under regal hardwoods to end at 2.1 miles. From there it is a quarter-mile downhill back to the primary trailhead near the Hillman Ferry gatehouse.

■ HILLMAN HERITAGE TRAIL: Vogle Loop

TYPE Bicycle and foot   **DIFFICULTY** Moderate   **LENGTH** 1.0 mile
USE Moderate   **CONDITION** Good
HIGHLIGHTS Vogle homesite, lake views, quarry sites
CONNECTIONS Bohannon Loop

THE VOGLE LOOP is stretched out on a peninsula and arguably provides more highlights than any other trail in the Hillman Heritage network. It leaves the Bohannon Loop about a mile from the Hillman Ferry gatehouse trailhead, then heads south, coming to a sharp slope above an old quarry, partly submerged by Kentucky Lake. User-created trails head to outcrops above the quarry. The scenic outcrops are known to attract partiers from the lake but are worth a visit nonetheless. Beyond there, the Vogle Loop drops to the lake's edge and stone remnants of the Vogle homesite. The Vogle family started Star Lime Works prior to the Civil War and was largely responsible for this community coming to be. Just beyond here, the trail drops to a gravel bar with an extensive lake panorama. Beyond this, climb past a limestone mine access used by the Tennessee Valley Authority. The mine access is gated off. From here, you rise through hackberry groves along a bluff above the lake on a narrow path. Join the top of a dry quarry to your right before dropping to pass a spur leading left to a cove and lake beach. Finally, return to meet the Bohannon Loop at 1.0 mile.

■ HILLMAN HERITAGE TRAIL: Brown Spring Loop

TYPE Bicycle and foot   **DIFFICULTY** Moderate   **LENGTH** 0.7 mile
USE High   **CONDITION** Good, steep section
HIGHLIGHTS Good for Hillman Ferry campers   **CONNECTIONS** Connectors

THE BROWN SPRING LOOP is a short circuit often used by Hillman Ferry campers to make a little loop from near the campground boat ramp. It is most easily accessed from near this boat ramp where it rises to a connector leading left to the Bohannon Loop. Going counterclockwise, the trail then heads south along a hardwood-clad ridge to meet a 0.1-mile connector linking it to the James Nickell Loop. The path then turns north and makes a long, steep descent before hitting a low point only to climb and finish its 0.7-mile loop.

■ HILLMAN HERITAGE TRAIL: James Nickell Loop

TYPE Bicycle and foot   **DIFFICULTY** Moderate   **LENGTH** 0.5 mile
USE High   **CONDITION** Good
HIGHLIGHTS Kentucky Lake vista   **CONNECTIONS** Connectors

THE JAMES NICKELL LOOP is best known for the superlative overlook at its most southerly point. Accessed via a combination of connectors and the Brown

Spring Loop, it first traces an old road south atop a hill then drops to a grassy point, mixed with a few hickories. Here, the prominence above Kentucky Lake allows extensive views—both south down the reach of the impoundment as well as across water. This is a view not to be missed. From the vista, the path roller coasters along the edge of a drop-off, then returns to its point of origin at 0.5 mile.

ACCESS From the North Welcome Station, head south on Woodlands Trace for 1.5 miles to Forest Road 110. Turn right on FR 110 and follow it to dead-end at the Hillman Ferry Campground gatehouse. The trail parking is on the right just before the gatehouse. The trail network begins on the far side of the gatehouse.

Central Hardwoods Scenic Trail

THE CENTRAL HARDWOODS SCENIC TRAIL is a fantastic addition to an already well-developed trail system at LBL. This trail makes an east–west track across the entirety of the LBL peninsula, running roughly parallel to US 68/KY 80. The trail is open to hikers and bicyclers but is primarily used by the two-wheeled set. The grades are gentle, making it doable by hikers and bicyclers of all capabilities. Streams are bridged or crossed via culvert. The route is more similar to a rail-trail than it is a mountain biking trail, though elevation changes are common, and the path is steeper than a rail-trail. In fact, elevation changes stretch a little over 200 feet between the lakes and the ridgetops around Golden Pond. The trail builders did a spectacular job grading the path to make the elevation changes doable by your average bicycler. Covering 11 miles one way from the Fenton trailhead near Kentucky Lake to the Cumberland trailhead near Lake Barkley, the Central Hardwoods Scenic Trail winds through woods, along ridges, and across drainages. The trail surface is mostly compact gravel, save for the east end, which is paved. Multiple trailheads make doing varied stretches of the path a breeze. The path is often started at the Golden Pond Visitor Center, though its official beginning is Fenton and runs east to Lake Barkley. Camping is not allowed on the trail. A trail map is available at Golden Pond Visitor Center and online.

■ **CENTRAL HARDWOODS SCENIC TRAIL:**
Fenton to Cumberland

TYPE Bicycle and foot   **DIFFICULTY** Moderate   **LENGTH** 11 miles
USE High   **CONDITION** Good
HIGHLIGHTS Lake views, wildflowers, fall colors   **CONNECTIONS** North–South Trail

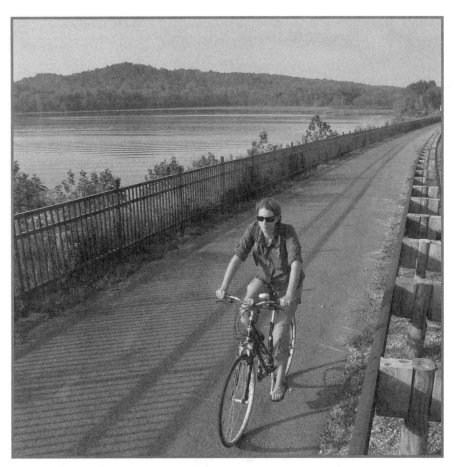

Central Hardwoods Scenic Trail near Devils Elbow

THE CENTRAL HARDWOODS TRAIL leaves east from a road just beyond the Fenton Picnic Shelter. A kiosk displays a trail map and information. Join the compacted gravel track as it rises from fields to pass an interpretive sign describing a former fishing camp—Fisherman's One Stop—that once occupied the locale a century back. Rise into a forest of oak, cedar, hickory, maple, and sassafras. The path quickly joins and leaves a roadbed. Though heading uphill, the grade is gentle as you rise, curving in and out of coves, passing more former settler roads. By 1.0 mile, you have gained 200 feet. From here, the trail more or less levels off, gently undulating into hollows and rising slightly onto hills. Almost the whole trail is shaded in this segment. Pass occasional repose benches. Watch for sharp turns and occasional gravel washouts. At 1.6 miles, bridge a pair of streambeds, then join a doubletrack, an old road. Pass the Lee Cemetery on your left. Skirt forest and field, then come to the English Hill Trailhead at 2.0 miles. This signed trailhead is accessed by a short spur off US 68/KY 80.

The next segment of the Central Hardwoods Scenic Trail goes from English Hill to Golden Pond Visitor Center. Leave English Hill and head east, skirting the upper reaches of the Turkey Creek watershed. White oaks are prevalent here. At 2.6 miles, emerge onto an open area very near US 68/KY 80. Return to woods, crossing bridges at 2.7, 3.2, and 3.3 miles. The path winds and turns, crossing three more trail bridges at 3.5 and 3.6 miles. All those streams flow into Turkey Creek. Pass the intersection with the North–South Trail, cross one last bridge, then curve right to cross the main road of LBL, Woodlands Trace. Shortly arrive at the rear of Golden Pond Visitor Center at 4.0 miles.

The segment from Golden Pond Visitor Center to Meredith trailhead starts out by following an old asphalt path east and downhill, splitting left, then emerging at

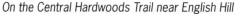

On the Central Hardwoods Trail near English Hill

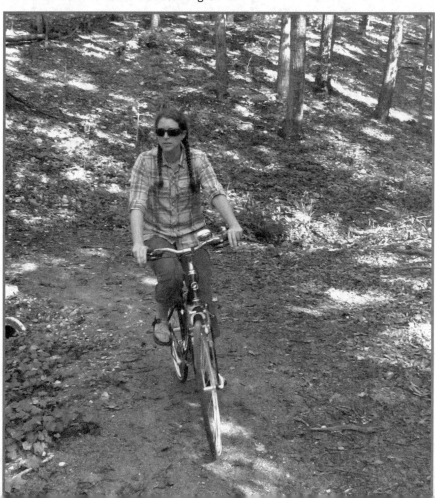

a dead end paved road. Head briefly left along the road, then right. These turns are signed. Join the customary compacted gravel track. Pass by some fields before entering a pine grove at 5.0 miles. At 5.6 miles, make a sharp curve left then bridge a tributary of Elbow Creek. Just ahead, cross a second bridge. Hollows drop off sharply in this area. At 6.1 miles, come to a trail intersection. Here a spur path leads left to the Meredith trailhead, reached off US 68/KY 80 via Forest Road 68/80-C.

The next segment from Meredith to Sunset trailhead involves a 200-foot descent, though it is gentle and well graded. From Meredith head east to crisscross old roads in a deciduous forest. Stay with the clearly identified compact gravel track. Pass under a power line at 6.7 miles. The descent continues and you enter an area of mixed field and forest, the site of the town of Golden Pond. At 7.7 miles, a spur leads left to an interpretive site concerning landowner plots at Golden Pond. Continue downhill in trees and grasses then reach a trail intersection at 8.0 miles. Here, a paved path leaves left 0.1 mile to tunnel under US 68/KY 80 and reach the Sunset trailhead and the end of this segment. The other way is the now-paved continuation of the Central Hardwoods Scenic Trail.

From Sunset, the paved path crosses FR 160, then comes along cultivated flats of Elbow Creek. Elevation changes are negligible beyond here, and the Central Hardwoods Scenic Trail seems more a rail-trail or urban greenway as it roughly parallels the highway next to it. There is little shade from here on out as well.

Bridge Elbow Creek at 8.3 and 8.8 miles. The travel is easy, but this segment is more suited for bicyclers than hikers. The Long Creek embayment of Lake Barkley comes into view by 9.0 miles. Share a causeway with US 68/KY 80 and open onto the embayment. Bridge Long Creek then come to the Devils Elbow trailhead at 10.0 miles. The actual parking area is below you, at the boat ramp.

The final segment of the Central Hardwoods Scenic Trail stretches from Devils Elbow to Lake Barkley. Leave Devils Elbow, running alongside the highway. Crest over a small hill, running parallel to US 68/KY 80 then open onto Lake Barkley and reach Lake Barkley at 11.0 miles, ending the Central Hardwoods Scenic Trail.

ACCESS   *West Access:* From the entrance of the Golden Pond Visitor Center, drive north to US 68/KY 80. Head west on US 68/KY 80 2.5 miles to the campground, on your left, just before the bridge over Kentucky Lake. Follow the access road toward the Fenton Picnic Shelter. Continue a little past the shelter to dead-end at the trailhead. *East Access:* The east access is on US 68/KY 80 just before the bridge over Lake Barkley.

Energy Lake Trails

A FIGURE-EIGHT DOUBLE LOOP TRAIL emanates from Energy Lake Campground. These trails are most often used by campers at Energy Lake, but are not exclusively for their use. The trails are hilly, but the vertical variation adds an exercise component to the attractive scenery of the lower Crooked Creek Valley. A trail map is available at the Energy Lake Campground entrance station and online.

■ LOOP 1

TYPE Foot only   **DIFFICULTY** Moderate   **LENGTH** 3.9 miles

USE Low   **CONDITION** Fair to good

HIGHLIGHTS Lake views, solitude   **CONNECTIONS** Connector Trail, Loop 2

THE ONLY THING the Energy Lake Trails lack is a creative name. The names "Loop 1" and "Loop 2" are unimaginative at best. The only reason the namers didn't use "Loop A" and "Loop B" is that these letters were already taken as part of Energy Lake Campground loops. Names aside, these trails offer Energy Lake campers and others a chance to stretch their legs along the perimeter of Crooked Creek Valley.

This is a good trail. It makes for a challenging hike as the path winds through remote hills, alongside Crooked Creek Bay, then Shaw Branch Bay, and back to Energy Lake Campground with the help of the Connector Trail. Being little used, the trail tread is not developed, making it hard to follow at times, although the path is well blazed. It also goes where you think it won't, or shouldn't, go, further complicating matters. And you won't likely run into anyone else in the area to ask for directions, at least away from Lake Barkley. All the above adds up to an intriguing hike worth two hours—or more if you get lost—of your time.

Start Loop 1 at the entrance gate to Energy Lake Campground. If you are not camping at Energy Lake, park your car on the shoulder of Forest Road 134 away from the campground. Walk on the road toward Energy Lake and look right for the blazed trail entering the woods from the shoulder of FR 134. Enter a hollow, then trace a faint roadbed up the hollow.

Curve away from the hollow, climbing to a hilltop and trail junction at 0.3 mile. Turn left here, staying with Loop 1, as the also-uninspiringly named Connector Trail leaves right. Descend the hilltop, then make an abrupt right turn, the first unexpected turn of Loop 1. The trail bed is indistinct here; stay with Loop 1 as it heads north for Energy Dam Day-Use Area at mile 1.0. The day-use area and FR 134 are visible through the trees. Turn right, walking along Crooked Creek Bay of Lake Barkley.

Begin to circle around a cove, crossing the streambed forming the cove. Loop 1 heads toward the lake, then turns right suddenly and directly away from the water. Reach a roadbed on a hill at mile 1.8. Turn right and follow the roadbed just a short distance. Fight the urge to continue on the roadbed, as the blue blazes lead left on a singletrack tread that dips down to Shaw Branch Bay. The trail is narrow and sloped. Come within sight of the bay before leaving the water and crossing the roadbed you left earlier. A field lies to your left.

Keep forward, crossing a small streambed. Curve around to the right as FR 134 comes into view to your left. Turn left abruptly to reach FR 134. You think the trail will resume directly across the forest road, but it doesn't. Turn left on the forest road and look for Loop 1 reentering the woods on the far side of FR 134. It shortly passes a homesite once shaded by a huge white oak with widespread branches.

You are now in Boardinghouse Hollow. Many residents lived in what was known as Between The Rivers long before the Tennessee and Cumberland were dammed, long before the Tennessee Valley Authority purchased the land, and long before the U.S. Forest Service came to manage this recreation area. Roads were poor and stores were few. Residents often bought goods from men who drove trucks and made the rounds of these forgotten hollows, selling everything from perfume to hoes.

Loop 1 ascends away from the homesite to make a ridgeline. Cruise the ridge and come to FR 146 and a power line. Turn left on the road and march a few steps, then turn right back into the woods. Shortly, meet the Connector Trail at mile 3.2. Loop 1 turns right onto the yellow-blazed Connector Trail and passes back under the power line. Descend to again cross FR 134. Climb away from the gravel road to meet a trail junction. You have been here before. Turn left, leaving the Connector Trail and descend to reach the Energy Lake Campground entrance gate.

ACCESS   From the North Welcome Station, take Woodlands Trace south 9.0 miles to FR 133, Silver Trail Road. Turn left on Silver Trail Road and follow it 3.0 miles to FR 134. Turn right on FR 134 and follow it 4.5 miles to Energy Lake Campground. The blue-blazed trail starts across from campground entrance, just a little toward Energy Lake.

■ **LOOP 2**

TYPE Foot only   **DIFFICULTY** Moderate   **LENGTH** 2.1 miles
USE Moderate   **CONDITION** Good
HIGHLIGHTS Convenient loop trail passing directly through campground
CONNECTIONS Connector Trail, Loop 1

START LOOP 2 at the entrance gate to Energy Lake Campground. If you are not camping at Energy Lake, park your car on the shoulder of Forest Road 134 away from the campground. Walk on the road toward Energy Lake and look right for the blue-blazed trail entering the woods from the shoulder of FR 134. Enter a hollow, then trace a faint roadbed up the hollow. The trail was formerly marked with red paint blazes on the trees, which are still visible.

Curve away from the hollow, climbing to a hilltop and trail junction at 0.3 mile. Turn right here, now on the Connector Trail. Loop 1 leaves left here. Loop 2 takes the Connector Trail right, which curves around the top of a knob and descends to cross FR 134 at 0.6 mile.

Climb through an open area growing up in winged elm. This tree with the unusual name often grows in abandoned clearings. Winged elms are easily identified by the corky "wings" running along their branches. The fiber-like inner bark of this tree was made into a rope and used to tie cotton bales in the 1800s. Winged elms are commonly seen in LBL. Look for winged elms on the perimeter of ridgetop clearings that are becoming reforested.

The canopy soon closes over the Connector Trail. Reach another junction at 0.7 mile. Turn right here, rejoining Loop 2. The trail becomes rutted as it dips toward an unnamed streambed flowing into Energy Lake. The flat widens and just as you think the trail is leading to Energy Lake, it turns up a hill, then begins to parallel the impoundment along a slope. Energy Lake holds back the waters of Crooked Creek. Head toward Energy Campground, passing alongside an old wire fence. Notice where the fence has grown into trees in places.

Reach a shelter house of Energy Lake Campground at 1.7 miles, entering the campground at site D-9. Turn right here, leaving Area D and tracing the gravel campground road. Pass entrances to the camping loops C, B, A, and the campground swim beach. Complete Loop 2 after passing the campground gatehouse.

ACCESS From the North Welcome Station, take Woodlands Trace south 9.0 miles to FR 133, Silver Trail Road. Turn left on Silver Trail Road and follow it 3.0 miles to FR 134. Turn right on FR 134 and follow it 4.5 miles to Energy Lake Campground. The trail starts across from the campground entrance, just a little toward Energy Lake.

Fort Donelson National Battlefield Trails

FORT DONELSON NATIONAL BATTLEFIELD is a separate federal entity just south of Land Between The Lakes National Recreation Area. It was at this Civil War site that the Union army began chiseling a wedge through the heart of the Confederacy, ultimately splitting it in two. The Confederacy had built forts protecting the mouths of the Tennessee and Cumberland Rivers. The Union first attacked and overwhelmed Fort Henry, located inside today's Land Between The Lakes boundaries. The Confederates retreated to Fort Donelson. The Union followed and began surrounding the rebels, who had hastily constructed an outer perimeter of earthworks to protect Fort Donelson. Seeing the futility of their position, the rebels cleared an escape route up the Cumberland and left. Others were left to defend the fort and surrendered to Union general Ulysses S. Grant. This battle was the first step from obscurity to the presidency for the general.

Today, the battlefield is preserved. The trails are just one way to visit the battlefield. Visitors can also tour by auto, seeing the Confederate Memorial, National Cemetery, earthworks, and cannon emplacements overlooking the Cumberland River. Interpretive information has been added around the battlefield for a better understanding of what occurred on that February of 1862. Before you hike any of the trails at Fort Donelson, be sure to stop at the visitor center to peruse their interpretive information too.

ACCESS Fort Donelson Visitor Center is located near Dover, Tennessee, 1.5 miles east of Woodlands Trace on US 79 South.

■ DONELSON TRAIL

TYPE Foot only   **DIFFICULTY** Moderate   **LENGTH** 3.1 miles
USE Moderate   **CONDITION** Good
HIGHLIGHTS Makes a loop through most of Fort Donelson's historic features
CONNECTIONS River Circle Trail, Spur Trail

THE HISTORICAL IMPORTANCE of the trailside setting is obvious, but the beauty of the setting will surprise hikers. Travel along flanks of Confederate earthworks, erected to protect Fort Donelson, which guarded the lower Cumberland River. Pass a tall monument to Confederate soldiers. Drop into and climb out of steep wooded ravines that were a factor in the strategic locating of Fort Donelson. Next, reach the shores of Lake Barkley and come to the actual fort, where river batteries look over a stunning sweep of the Cumberland River. Visit log hut replicas that housed Confederate troops. Enjoy a woods walk while returning to the visitor center and completing the loop.

The trail begins near the 6-pound cannon at the entrance to visitor center parking area. A sign states DONELSON TRAIL, 3.1 MILES. In other places, the trail is denoted with a brown sign and a hiker symbol on it. Turn right as you face the sign and begin walking a mown path. The Confederate earthworks to your right were trenches that protected soldiers. The hillside drops steeply to your left. Johnny Reb set up these earthworks using the steep terrain as an added measure of defense. The Union would have had to ascend the hills and storm the trenches to breach this outer perimeter. The mixture of scattered trees, grass, and woods belies this area's violent past. Shortly, reach the Confederate Monument on your right. This tall stone pillar is topped with a metal Confederate soldier in uniform. Return to the trail and keep north along the rebel trenches, soon passing the site of Smith's attack. Union forces under General C. F. Smith captured these earthworks. Ahead is the site of Jackson's Battery, a Confederate position later abandoned when the rebels decided to break for Nashville.

Reach a trail junction at 0.5 mile. To the left is the River Circle Trail, which makes a good loop when combined with the Donelson Trail. The Donelson Trail enters the woods, uphill and to the right of the River Circle Trail, and soon descends by switchbacks into a deep and steep hollow through which an intermittent stream flows. The moss-bed trail climbs past a triple-trunked beech tree before making a field atop a hill. Look to your right and see three old, gnarled tulip trees that were once part

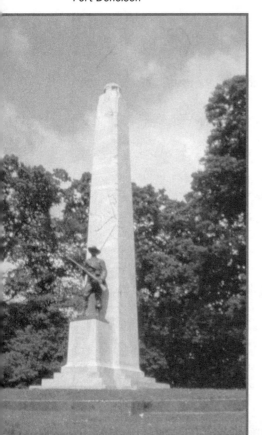

Confederate Memorial at Fort Donelson

of a homestead. Keep forward, pass a withering stock pond, and dive into a second hollow, crossing a gullied streambed. Begin to head downstream above the main hollow. Big tulip trees shade the ravine. The hollow opens and meets the River Circle Trail at mile 1.6.

Stay right on the Donelson Trail and soon come out at the Upper River Battery. Here, Confederates used heavy artillery to bombard Union ironclad gunboats into withdrawing. It is easy to see that these well-placed cannons could control the Cumberland River at this point. What you see today is Lake Barkley, since the Cumberland is dammed downstream.

The trail becomes hard to follow here. Leave the river batteries and climb uphill on the road toward two log huts. These replicas are like those that housed Confederate soldiers but were burned down to fight a measles outbreak after the Union took over. Turn left on the road that leads to the "Luncheon

Area." This is the first time I have seen a picnic area referred to on a sign as a "Luncheon Area." Anyway, make the picnic area, looking for a huge oak tree backed by earthworks. The trail picks up again here, descending to a ravine along earthworks (look for a hiker symbol on a small brown sign). The path is mown as it passes through an open field. Soon, reenter woods, heading south, and climb to enter a thick pine grove. At mile 2.6, make a sharp left onto an old roadbed. Pass through low woods before leaving right from the roadbed and climbing to another pine grove.

At mile 2.9, reach a trail junction. Here, the Spur Trail leads left 1.3 miles to the Fort Donelson National Cemetery. The Donelson Trail turns right in south-facing hickory-oak woods, then dives into a ravine. Cross an intermittent streambed on a footbridge, then climb out of the ravine by switchbacks. Shortly, reach the back side of the visitor center and complete the loop.

ACCESS   The Donelson Trail starts near the cannon to your left, as you are looking out from the Fort Donelson National Battlefield Visitor Center.

■ EARTHWORKS TRAIL

TYPE Foot only   **DIFFICULTY** Easy to moderate   **LENGTH** 1.3 miles
USE Too low   **CONDITION** Good
HIGHLIGHTS Connects battlefield visitor center with national cemetery
CONNECTIONS Donelson Trail

THIS LITTLE-USED AND UNDERRATED PATH at Fort Donelson National Battlefield traverses a corridor of protected land. The trail runs parallel to Confederate earthworks nearly its entire distance. Along the way, it passes over three sizable hills, on top of which were artillery batteries connected by these earthworks.

If you tour Fort Donelson, take the time to also hike this path—it needs some feet on it. Before you hike it though, stop at the visitor center and get acquainted with the battle. Fort Donelson and nearby Fort Henry were built by the rebels to hold sway over the Tennessee and Cumberland Rivers. This way the Union couldn't use the waterways for troop or supply movements. Fort Henry was poorly located in a low area subject to flooding by the Tennessee River. In February 1863, it was easily bombed into submission by Federal ironclad gunboats. The rebels escaped easterly to Fort Donelson, well located on a hill with a sweeping view of the Cumberland River. The soldiers of Fort Henry reached Fort Donelson, already protected by earthworks, then built an outer perimeter of trenches beyond the fort. These earthworks were stretched along high ground from Hickman Creek in the west to the tiny town of Dover in the east. The earthworks you follow on this trail were part of the outer perimeter.

Federal gunboats couldn't do much against the well-placed rebel artillery at Fort Donelson, but while the water war was going on, Federal troops were amassing around the whole rebel perimeter. The Union crashed the perimeter, but the rebels pushed them back. In the confusion of battle, the rebels were ordered to return to their original positions behind the earthworks. The Union attacked again and retook the territory they had lost and gained some to boot. Finally, most Confederates escaped southeasterly to Nashville, leaving a few to defend Fort Donelson, which was surrendered to General Grant the next day.

While you are hiking, imagine Confederate and Union troops poised on either side of the earthworks beside you. Leave the circular parking area and head downhill on the grassy part of the corridor. A cannon representing Graves Battery is to your right. A small brown hiker sign leads the way downhill. The mown field is cut a little lower along the barely discernible trail. Dive off the hill to reach a wooded flat on your left. The earthworks are to your right. Cross a quaint little bridge over Indian Creek, a clear stream. Keep forward beyond the bridge through a field flanked on the left by cedar trees.

Reach Sandy Road and continue forward. An interpretive sign about the activities of Nathan Bedford Forrest stands to your left. Ascend the wooded hill ahead of you. It is easy to see the narrowness of this protected corridor, as houses are visible

River batteries at Fort Donelson

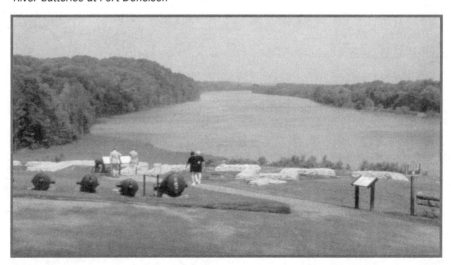

nearby. Tall cedar and oak trees shade the route. The earthworks remain to your right. Head up the steep hill and top out at the location of Maney's Battery. The rebels smartly picked this hilltop with its potential views. Trees were felled back then to open points of observation and clear lines of fire. This four-cannon unit was placed here along with French's Battery on the next hill to keep the Union from sneaking down Erin Hollow, where you are headed, to attack Fort Donelson.

Turn left at Maney's Battery, now descending again on a long hill. The rebel trenches remain to your right. Shortly, arrive at the bottom of Erin Hollow. Span the intermittent stream on a wooden bridge. The trail here becomes a bit obscure, but begin climbing uphill, keeping the earthworks to your right.

The trail opens in a field and climbs steeply to the third hill. Atop is a most attractive setting. Large hardwoods flank a level grassy area, the site of French's Battery. Interpretive signs tell the story of what happened. Ahead is a small parking area and Cedar Street, and the end of this trail. Your best bet is to retrace your steps back to Graves Battery.

ACCESS From the Fort Donelson Visitor Center, turn left on US 79, heading 0.1 mile back toward Dover. Turn right onto an unnamed paved road and follow it a short distance to dead-end at the location of Graves Battery. The trail follows the field downhill as you look toward the cannon at Graves Battery.

■ RIVER CIRCLE TRAIL

TYPE Foot only   **DIFFICULTY** Easy to moderate   **LENGTH** 1.1 miles
USE Low to moderate   **CONDITION** Good
HIGHLIGHTS Combine this trail with part of Donelson Trail for a good loop, lake views, wildflowers in spring   **CONNECTIONS** Donelson Trail

THIS TRAIL IS RECOMMENDED as one half of a loop hike. The trail description heads from east to west, as it is most often hiked. Hikers will be surprised at the steepness of this trail as it crosses ravines running up the hill atop which Fort Donelson sits.

From the east junction with the Donelson Trail, near the river batteries, pass along the Hickman Creek embayment, part of Lake Barkley. When the battle was fought, Hickman Creek flowed free into the Cumberland River. Turn into a ravine. Just before spanning a bridge over the ravine, look left for a rocked-in spring that may have provided water for soldiers of the battle.

Climb out of the desiccated hollow and come near a field, only to descend again, working around a narrow, steep ravine. Come again to Hickman Creek embayment, running alongside the water, pick up an intermittent streambed and follow it, roughly, away from the embayment up the hill to reach the parking turnaround near Jackson's Battery.

ACCESS From the Fort Donelson Visitor Center, continue into the battlefield, then veer left at the Confederate Monument. Follow this road down to a paved circle near Jackson's Battery. The River Circle Trail starts at the lower end of the grassy area by the pavement.

■ SPUR TRAIL

TYPE Foot only   **DIFFICULTY** Easy   **LENGTH** 1.3 miles
USE Low   **CONDITION** Good
HIGHLIGHTS Connects battlefield visitor center with national cemetery
CONNECTIONS Donelson Trail

THIS TRAIL LEAVES from the Fort Donelson National Cemetery and roams through woods to reach the main area of Fort Donelson National Battlefield. The cemetery grounds are thought provoking. A small visitor information building is staffed for answers to questions.

Start the Spur Trail by passing through the wrought iron cemetery gates and staying to the right of the battlefield cemetery. You may wish to see some of the memorials. Keep along the low wall to the right of the graves and look for concrete steps going over the low wall beside a large cedar tree. The trail descends a grassy area to veer left into woodland. Private property is to your right.

Circle around shady hardwood hollow. You can see the Cumberland River through the trees to your right. At 0.3 mile, the Spur Trail makes a sharp left by a contemplation bench. The path—marked with brown hiker signs at major turns— then heads up along the Indian Creek embayment. Occasional large hardwoods grow overhead. Descend to step over a wet-weather drainage very near the embayment. Look for the large multitrunked sycamore here. Pass through a clearing and open-air amphitheater. Watery views open to your right. Open onto Church Street and veer right on the grassy lane. Come directly alongside US 79 as the Spur Trail skirts the upper end of Indian Creek embayment.

Leave the road and climb by switchback to reach a trail junction at 1.3 miles. From here, the Donelson Loop leaves left to shortly reach the visitor center and right to reach the picnic area.

ACCESS From the Fort Donelson Visitor Center turn left, heading south on US 79. Follow it 0.7 mile to Church Street. Turn left on Church Street and follow it 0.3 mile to the left turn into the cemetery parking area. The Spur Trail starts past the wrought iron gates.

Fort Henry Area Trails

THE FORT HENRY TRAIL SYSTEM is concentrated in the southwest end of LBL. The entire system is a designated National Recreation Trail. A total of 30 miles comprise the trail system. To keep hikers oriented, numbered trail signs are located at trail junctions. These numbers are referred to as "points." For example, the junction where the Piney Trail and the Volunteer Trail meet is Point 21. A sign with the number 21 is posted at the junction, and the number 21 is shown on the official LBL Hike & Bike Trail Map. Obtain a trail map at either the welcome center or the main visitor center.

■ ARTILLERY TRAIL

TYPE Foot only   **DIFFICULTY** Moderate   **LENGTH** 3.2 miles
USE Low to moderate   **CONDITION** Good
HIGHLIGHTS Traces Civil War route of Ulysses S. Grant, loop possibilities
CONNECTIONS Telegraph Trail, Piney Trail, Devils Backbone Trail, Peytona Trail

THIS TRAIL FOLLOWS part of a historic wagon road that reached from Fort Henry on the Tennessee River to Fort Donelson on the Cumberland River. The Artillery Trail is an interior trail and can only be reached via other paths, but the north end of the trail lies close to Fort Henry Road, making it easily accessible.

The Artillery Trail leaves south from the Telegraph Trail and mostly climbs to meet Picket Road, part of a historic route used by Grant. It then undulates along a ridgeline, topping out on Pine Hill, a high point, and keeps southeasterly to meet the Piney Trail, also on a ridgeline. From here, the trail curves east and soon meets the Devils Backbone Trail. Beyond this junction, the Artillery Trail cruises along a ridgetop through hickory, oak, and pine woods, passing a homesite along the way to meet the Peytona Trail, its culmination, within earshot of US 79.

Start the yellow-blazed Artillery Trail by leaving south from the Telegraph Trail at Point 4. Undulate along the ridgeline after reaching Picket Road at 0.3 mile, part of one historic route taken by Grant and his men heading toward Fort Donelson. The other route to Fort Donelson traveled along what is now the Telegraph Trail.

This ridgetop road the Artillery Trail follows, not much more than a wagon track, soon became muddy, gullied, and nearly impassable during early February of 1862. The Confederates were counting on the rough terrain between Fort Henry and Fort Donelson to slow the Union. Weather delayed the Union attack but didn't save Fort Donelson.

The ridgeline narrows and drops off on both sides as you reach Pine Hill at mile 1.0. Hickory, oak, and pine cloak the ridgeline. Moderately ascend for the last 0.2 mile, veering left at the end to meet the Piney Trail and Point 20 at mile 1.4. From here, the Piney Trail leaves right for 2.3 miles to reach Piney Campground. The Artillery Trail veers left and continues southeasterly along a nearly level ridge with mixed pines and oaks. Before you know it, the Artillery Trail reaches Point 18 and the Devils Backbone Trail at mile 1.6. The Devils Backbone Trail leaves left for 1.5 miles to meet the Telegraph Trail. The Artillery Trail heads on to an isolated divide separating Panther Creek to your left and Lost Creek to your right. You are likely to hear nothing but the wind blowing through the trees atop this quiet high line.

At mile 2.1, the canopy opens. Reach a clearing in varied stages of regrowth. To your left is an obvious old homesite shaded by a large oak and some large sugar maples, which were often planted in yards of former residents. Most of the old-growth trees you see in LBL are remnants of those planted long ago by those who settled near them. Look around for other evidence of settlement. The Artillery Trail continues in brushy woods.

Resume walking among shortleaf pines and varied oaks. Leave the pines at mile 2.7 and continue in hardwoods for the easy last half mile, reaching Point 17 and the Peytona Trail at mile 3.2. From here, the Peytona Trail leaves left for 0.7 mile to meet the Tennessee Ridge Trail. An access road keeps forward for 0.1 mile to meet US 79.

ACCESS The Artillery Trail is an interior trail. The quickest access is to take the Picket/Telegraph Trail from Point 26 on Fort Henry Road 0.3 mile to meet the Telegraph Trail. Take the Telegraph Trail east 0.2 mile to reach the northwest end of the Artillery Trail. Access from US 79 is discouraged.

■ BOSWELL TRAIL

TYPE Foot only **DIFFICULTY** Easy **LENGTH** 0.4 mile
USE Moderate **CONDITION** Good
HIGHLIGHTS Connects Boswell Landing Lake Access to Picket Loop Trail
CONNECTIONS Picket Loop Trail

VISITORS TO BOSWELL LANDING LAKE ACCESS use this yellow-blazed path to reach the 2.2-mile Picket Loop Trail. Adding the out-and-back distance of the Boswell Trail makes the total mileage for Boswell/Picket Loop 3.0 miles. The Boswell Trail runs alongside Forest Road 233 a bit, then veers east, crossing a couple of intermittent streambeds to meet the Picket Loop at Point 24.

Start this hike behind picnic/campsite 2 atop the hill at Boswell Landing Lake Access. Head away from the lake and meander alongside FR 233, turning east. Shortly, reach a streambed in a steep ravine. Step over this normally dry ravine then dip to an old, wide roadbed. Cross this roadbed and step over one more dry branch to meet the Picket Loop Trail at 0.4 mile. This is Point 24. From here, turn left and it is 1.2 miles to the Picket Loop trailhead and Point 26 and 0.5 mile to Point 23, also on the Picket Loop Trail.

ACCESS From the South Welcome Station, take FR 230, Fort Henry Road, 4.1 miles to FR 232. Turn right on FR 232 and follow it 0.1 mile to FR 233. Turn right on FR 233 and follow it 1.2 miles to dead-end at the landing. The Boswell Trail starts near picnic/campsite 2, by the Campbell Cemetery. Look for a sign indicating POINT 25 on a tree.

■ DEVILS BACKBONE TRAIL

TYPE Foot only   **DIFFICULTY** Moderate   **LENGTH** 1.5 miles
USE Moderate   **CONDITION** Good   **HIGHLIGHTS** Knife-edge ridge, pretty valley
CONNECTIONS Telegraph Trail, Artillery Trail

THIS IS ONE of the best trails in the Fort Henry Trail System. When combined with the Artillery Trail it makes a quality loop. The Devils Backbone Trail heads north from the Artillery Trail along an ever-narrowing ridgeline until hikers can see simultaneously into Buckingham Hollow to the west and an unnamed hollow to the east. Finally, the ridge gives way and meets the stream draining the two hollows in attractive bottomland before meeting the Telegraph Trail.

Leave Point 18 and the Artillery Trail, heading northeast in level woods on the blue-blazed Devils Backbone Trail. Shortly, the trail reaches Point 19. The Devils Backbone Trail stays left and descends in hickory, oak, and pine woods. The ridgeline continues to get lower and narrower as hollows develop on both sides of the path. Look on the trail's left for an unusual tree that makes a natural bench—it grows vertically for a foot, then horizontally for a couple of feet, then back to vertically.

The rocky path shifts to the west side of the ridge at 0.5 mile. You can look off this steep bluff into Buckingham Hollow. Keep an eye out for mountain laurel growing on the side of this bluff. This plant likely migrated down the Tennessee River from the Southern Appalachians where it is found in abundance. It is very rare in the Cumberland River drainage.

Keep descending as the Devils Backbone becomes rocky and narrows to the point where you can see into both Buckingham Hollow and the hollow to the east. The ridgeline is hardly wider than the trail itself. By mile 1.2, the Devils Backbone has petered out and the path enters a large flat created by the two hollows merging into one. Cross the streambed coming from Buckingham Hollow and enter an attractive area of mixed cedars and hardwoods growing alongside the combined streambed, now flowing perennially from an upstream spring. At mile 1.5, reach Point 5 and the Telegraph Trail. The Devils Backbone Trail ends here. The Telegraph Trail leaves right to span a wooden bridge and reach the Fort Henry trailhead.

ACCESS The Devils Backbone Trail is an interior trail. The quickest access is to follow the Telegraph Trail west from Point 7 in the Fort Henry Trail System for 0.4 mile to reach the north end of the Devils Backbone Trail.

■ PEYTONA TRAIL

TYPE Foot only   **DIFFICULTY** Moderate   **LENGTH** 3.0 miles
USE Moderate   **CONDITION** Good   **HIGHLIGHTS** Beaver dams, homesites
CONNECTIONS Telegraph Trail, Tennessee Ridge Trail, Artillery Trail

THE PEYTONA TRAIL heads up the watershed of Bear Creek, passing fields and homesites. Where there once were human residents, beavers have taken over, making dams and ponds. The Peytona Trail leaves Bear Creek and heads for Tennessee Ridge, one of the higher points at LBL. The end of the trail leaves Tennessee Ridge and descends to Lick Hollow, a pretty valley full of wildflowers. It then climbs back onto the next ridge where it meets the Artillery Trail within earshot of US 79. The Peytona Trail is named for the nearby Peytona Furnace, operated by Thomas Kirkman. He named his furnace after a famous racehorse of 1845. The furnace was temporarily rendered inoperable by Federal troops immediately after the Battle of Fort Donelson.

Leave the Telegraph Trail at Point 11. Immediately cross the Dry Branch streambed and enter a field. Circle around the right side of the field before reentering woods at the back of the field. Head south in second- or third-growth woodland, coming alongside Bear Creek. Check out the flat to your left for gnawed trees and beaver ponds.

At 0.5 mile, just beyond a homesite on your left with a wide-crowned sugar maple, the Peytona Trail leaves uphill away from the road, circling around beaver dams. Immediately pass a huge beech tree then the small Wofford Cemetery. Climb a hill, then return to the main trail bed. At mile 1.1, pass another homesite on your right. Look for concrete steps and a wire-encircled well. Look for the blue and black rocks in the trail bed. These are slag rocks, byproducts of the 1800s iron industry. This waste rock was often hauled away from furnace sites and used to gravel roads. Blue slag indicated high-grade iron ore, whereas black slag meant poorer ore. Keep forward and reach Point 15 at mile 1.3. Turn right, away from nearby US 79, and wind uphill toward Tennessee Ridge. Look around for remains of old cars. Though never overly steep, this hill continues on a moderate grade. An old road comes in on the left just as the trail levels off. Just ahead, reach Point 16 and the Tennessee Ridge Trail at mile 2.3.

At Point 16, the Peytona Trail veers left. The Tennessee Ridge Trail keeps forward 1.8 miles to meet the Telegraph Trail. Follow the Peytona Ridge Trail down a dry ridge replete with chestnut oak. Descend to cross a dry streambed twice and reach a low point at 2.6 miles. You are now in Lick Hollow. Veer upstream along another streambed. The streambeds of this hollow, when flowing, feed South Fork Panther Creek. Wildflowers abound in this north-facing cove in spring. Keep uphill along a low bluffline along the streambed. Pick up a finger ridge and soon reach Point 17 at 3.0 miles. The Peytona Trail ends here. A roadbed leads acutely left 0.1 mile to US 79. The Artillery Trail leaves right to meet the Devils Backbone Trail in 1.6 miles.

ACCESS The Peytona Trail is an interior trail. It can be reached by hiking the North–South Connector Trail 0.8 mile to the Telegraph Trail. Turn left on the Telegraph Trail and follow it 1.0 mile to reach the northeast end of the Peytona Trail. Access from US 79 is discouraged.

■ PICKET LOOP TRAIL

TYPE Foot only   **DIFFICULTY** Moderate   **LENGTH** 3.6 miles
USE Moderate   **CONDITION** Mostly good
HIGHLIGHTS Views of Kentucky Lake, old homesites
CONNECTIONS Telegraph Trail, Telegraph/Picket Trail, Boswell Trail

THIS TRAIL IS one of two trails departing from the main Fort Henry trailhead. The blue-blazed path descends to a hollow and crosses Forest Road 233. It then ascends a ridge to meet the loop part of the Picket Loop Trail. Travel a hardwood ridgeline, soon skirting Panther Bay on Kentucky Lake. Pass near old homesites while walking lakeside, then ascend to meet the Boswell Trail, coming from the Boswell Landing Lake Access. Cruise in woodland to finish the loop part of the trail and backtrack to the Fort Henry trailhead.

From the Fort Henry trailhead signboard, Point 1 in the Fort Henry Trail System, turn right and follow the blue-blazed path as it circles around the parking area. The Telegraph Trail leaves left. The Picket Loop Trail shortly picks up a roadbed at a sign stating HORSES AND MOTOR VEHICLES PROHIBITED. Veer left on this roadbed and descend to a hollow. Once in the hollow, veer right. Bottomland lies to your left. A mixture of pine and hardwoods such as shagbark hickory, beech, and dogwood grows above moss and ferns. The narrowed trail crosses paved FR 233 at 0.4 mile. Keep up the hollow to pick up a finger ridge. Reach a trail junction at 0.7 mile. This is Point 23. Here, the loop part of the trail begins. Turn right and follow a jeep track into a clearing, then come very near FR 230. Briefly turn away from the road, then reach it, at Point 26, at 1.2 miles. Here, the combined Telegraph/Picket Trail leads across the road 0.3 mile to reach the Telegraph Trail.

The Picket Loop Trail veers away from the paved road onto an old jeep track. Briefly parallel FR 230, then curve north away from the road. Reach a small wildlife clearing at 1.4 miles, then pass through a second small clearing. Keep along the ridgeline as Panther Bay comes into view through the trees on the right. Dry Fork Bay is soon visible too. At 1.9 miles, the Picket Loop veers left. The old jeep track leads forward a short distance to a homesite atop a hill. This piece of property would go for big bucks today. A wire fence surrounds a bricked-in well, and large trees shade the locale. Depressions in the earth nearby may have been rifle pits from part of Fort Henry.

Tennessee's governor at the onset of the Civil War commissioned Fort Henry to help protect the Tennessee River. Nearby Fort Donelson was to protect the Cumberland River and prevent Union soldiers and supplies from heading up the waterway. Fort Henry was poorly located, however, and was soon bombed into submission by Federal gunboats in February 6, 1862. The rebels mostly fled to Fort Donelson, leaving a small contingent at Fort Henry, which surrendered. Very little is left of Fort Henry today, most of it submerged beneath Kentucky Lake.

Return to the Picket Loop, which descends to Kentucky Lake, then turns left up an embayment. Shortly, pass another homesite. This one has a brick chimney and an old magnolia tree. Curve around the embayment and come to the streambed forming the embayment. This area is potentially confusing. Two sets of blazes cross the streambed and eventually meet again. The Picket Loop Trail keeps curving around the bay, then climbs a hill, passing another homesite on trail right. It is marked by large oak trees and scattered stones. Soon, meet the Boswell Trail and Point 24 at mile 2.4. The Boswell Trail leaves right 0.4 mile to Boswell Landing Lake Access.

The Picket Trail keeps forward along a level jeep track through young forest. The canopy is open overhead. The blue blazes lead right, off the roadbed, and pass a hole encircled with wire. It is either an oversized well or an undersized pond. A well is the better guess. Rejoin the jeep track and meet Point 23 at mile 2.9. The nonloop part of the trail leaves right. Backtrack 0.7 mile to reach the Fort Henry trailhead. The Telegraph/Picket Trail leaves across the road to meet the Telegraph Trail in 0.3 mile.

ACCESS From the South Welcome Station, take FR 230, Fort Henry Road, 4.1 miles to FR 232. Turn right on FR 232 and follow it 0.1 mile, then keep forward as FR 232 turns to gravel and continues 0.2 mile farther to dead-end at a turnaround. Look on the west side for a trail signboard. Turn right at the signboard, following the blue-blazed path starting at a cedar tree.

■ PINEY TRAIL

TYPE Foot only   **DIFFICULTY** Moderate   **LENGTH** 2.3 miles
USE Moderate   **CONDITION** Good
HIGHLIGHTS Connects Piney Campground to Fort Henry Trail System
CONNECTIONS Volunteer Trail, Artillery Trail

THIS PATH OFFERS both lowland and ridgetop environments. It also passes a small cemetery and meets the historic route used by Ulysses S. Grant when his Federal troops marched from Fort Henry to Fort Donelson. From near the Piney Campground entrance, this trail heads east through small watersheds to reach South Fork Piney Creek and the Volunteer Trail. From the creek, it climbs a piney ridge with winter views of the surrounding ridges to meet the Artillery Trail—Grant's route.

Start the hike by climbing the grassy hill at the Piney Campground entrance road junction and look for a trail sign indicating Point 22, a marker in the Fort Henry Trail System. To your right are rusty parts of an old jalopy. Look left for the Rowlette Cemetery. It has but one grave marker. The Piney Trail traces red rectangular metal blazes through hickory-oak woods. Descend into a bottom carved with streambeds. Maple, beech, and sweet gum thrive down here. Step over the streambeds and climb toward a gap, passing a small wildlife pond. Split the gap at 0.5 mile and descend to a larger streambed. Cross this rocky watercourse and pick up a wagon road flanked by wire fences. The road passes by large hilltop oaks, indicating former homesteads, before descending again into the South Fork Piney Creek watershed. Soon, step over South

Fork Piney Creek. Keep forward to reach Point 21 at mile 1.3, where the yellow-blazed Volunteer Trail leaves left 2.2 miles to meet the Telegraph Trail. Infantry Pass Spring and its backcountry campsite lie up the hollow to your right. The Piney Trail continues east, leaving the creek and ascending a narrow ridgeline.

A mixture of shortleaf pines and oaks cloaks the steep-sided ridge. A real sense of remoteness falls over the east-running high line. The path meanders along, leveling off at around 600 feet in elevation. The walking is easy, and the Piney Trail soon reaches Point 20 at mile 2.3. Here, the Artillery Trail leaves left 1.4 miles to meet the Telegraph Trail.

ACCESS   From the South Welcome Station, take Forest Road 230, Fort Henry Road, 7.8 miles to the Piney Campground entrance road. To your left, up the hill, is the Piney Trail. Stay left, driving past the trailhead and campground entrance road, and look for a grassy parking area on the left near an auto sign that states PINEY CAMP-GROUND, WELCOME STATION 8.

■ TELEGRAPH TRAIL

TYPE Foot only   **DIFFICULTY** Moderate to difficult   **LENGTH** 7.5 miles
USE Moderate   **CONDITION** Good
HIGHLIGHTS Longest trail in Fort Henry Trail System, beaver dams, springs, backcountry campsites
CONNECTIONS Picket Loop Trail, Volunteer Trail, Telegraph/Picket Trail, Artillery Trail, Devils Backbone Trail, Tennessee Ridge Trail, North–South Connector Trail, Peytona Trail, North–South Trail

JUDGING BY ALL of the above trail connections, the Telegraph Trail sounds like the backbone of the Fort Henry Trail System. And it is. This trail roughly traces an old telegraph line and accompanying road that connected Fort Henry with Fort Donelson. It leaves the Fort Henry trailhead and heads southeast to meet the Volunteer Trail at Fort Henry Branch. The path then turns east along Fort Henry Branch to meet three south-running trails in succession. Ahead, the Telegraph Trail drops to South Fork Panther Creek and Blue Spring. From here, it climbs then drops again into the Bear Creek watershed, where it forms one of LBL's classic day hikes, the Bear Creek Loop. Pass Kirkman's Camp backcountry campsite before reaching the South Welcome Station and meeting the North–South Trail.

While hiking this trail, imagine the days following the fall of the area to Federal troops, who occupied both Fort Henry and Fort Donelson. The path you're walking on led those Union forces to Fort Donelson. After both forts fell to the Union,

Confederate guerrillas continually cut the telegraph lines connecting the two forts, despite daily patrols by Union soldiers. Frightened citizens and slaves seeking freedom crowded around the forts in search of safety and shelter. Union soldiers combed the area, confiscating food and supplies from citizens. The whole area of what is now the south end of LBL was chaos and confusion. Today, the area offers peaceful solace from the high-paced civilized world.

Start the red-blazed Telegraph Trail as it curves around the Fort Henry trailhead and shortly crosses gravel Forest Road 232. Descend from the gravel road to bottomland and pass near relics from an old homesite on the right. Ascend a low hill to come alongside a field to your right. A wire fence borders the field. Curve around the field and descend to reach Fort Henry Branch in an often-flooded bottomland. Soon, reach Fort Henry Road and a concrete culvert where Fort Henry Branch flows under Fort Henry Road. Ascend to cross the road and immediately descend on steps to reach Point 2 at 0.4 mile. Here, the Volunteer Trail leaves right 2.2 miles over North Fork and South Fork Piney Creek to meet the Piney Trail. The Telegraph Trail curves left, winding amid a wide bottom where Fort Henry Branch splits into numerous ribbons, some flowing, some not. Walk a singletrack path through this wide maple, ash, and sweet gum bottom. Intermittent branches feed Fort Henry Branch. Skirt around a low bluff at 0.7 mile, soon returning to bottomland.

At mile 1.1, in the headwaters of Fort Henry Branch, reach Point 3. A field is in view here, and the yellow-blazed Telegraph/Picket Trail leaves left 0.3 mile to first reach Fort Henry Road and then the Picket Loop Trail. The Telegraph Trail leaves Fort Henry Branch, keeping east in hickory-oak forest with the field still in view to your left (north). Shortly, the Telegraph Trail reaches Point 4 at mile 1.3. At this point, the Artillery Trail leaves right 1.4 miles to reach the Piney Trail.

The Telegraph Trail continues working east, dropping to a desiccated ravine, then climbing onto a hill, only to drop again where it meets a streamlet and the edge of a field. Step over the streamlet and head downstream to reach Point 5 and the Devils Backbone Trail at mile 1.8. Here, the Devils Backbone Trail keeps forward 1.5 miles to meet the Artillery Trail. The Telegraph Trail turns left and spans the stream that drains Buckingham Hollow on a footbridge. Enter a field beyond the bridge. Skirt the edge of the field to reenter woods, now climbing, and reach Point 6 at mile 2.1.

The Telegraph Trail continues east to meet FR 400 and Point 7 at mile 2.2. Turn right and trace FR 400 as it undulates then levels off near a large field to the north. Look for a pond in the field. The gravel road ends at an earthen barrier. The Telegraph Trail continues beyond the barrier to span South Fork Panther Creek on a wooden bridge and reaches Point 8 at mile 2.7. This is an attractive streambed with tan rock bars and limestone outcrops. A partially wooded flat spreads out past the bridge.

The Telegraph Trail follows the clear branch formed by Blue Spring, ascending a small bluff. Soon, pass Boswell Cemetery 1 on your left. It has only one known grave. From the bluff, hikers can look over beaver dams that have periodically flooded and kept open the streamside. Ahead, span an intermittent streambed on a metal grate bridge. Ascend away from the watershed on an old eroded wagon track. Many chestnut oaks grow atop this ridge. In winter, higher Tennessee Ridge is visible to the southeast.

The nearly level ridgeline makes for easy walking, and before you know it, the Telegraph Trail has reached Point 9 and the Tennessee Ridge Trail at mile 4.0. The Telegraph Trail continues forward, passing a successional field (a formerly cleared space now reforesting) on the right, while the Tennessee Ridge Trail leads 1.8 miles south to meet the Peytona Trail. Make an easy track over a rolling ridge to meet the Fort Henry North–South Trail Connector and Point 10 at 4.3 miles. The connector leads left 1.4 miles to meet the North–South Trail.

The Telegraph Trail keeps forward along a rib ridge between two feeder streams of Dry Branch. Descend among cedars to reach a field and bottomland, curving along the field to come alongside Dry Branch. The lush streamside woods and bluffs of Dry Branch are an appealing contrast to the hilltop oak-hickory forest. Come alongside the bed of Dry Branch, then cross a feeder stream of Dry Branch. The Telegraph Trail then runs the margin of woods between Dry Branch and a field. At 5.3 miles, reach Point 11. Here, the Peytona Trail leaves south across the Dry Branch streambed.

The Telegraph Trail keeps forward alongside Bear Creek. A side trail leads left to a field just before the path crosses Bear Creek streambed. Keep along the creek beside a bluff and pass alongside a field and through a young, spindly forest to reach Point 12. Keep forward along the old road and reach Kirkman's Camp at mile 5.9. A fallen wood building, once a home, lies across the trail from the concreted spring. Thomas Kirkman received a land grant from the state of Tennessee in 1845. He built an iron furnace on land not far from this spring. It is hard to imagine the community that sprang up around the iron furnace among today's woods and fields. The community was short-lived however, as the Civil War interrupted production at the furnace. Like many other area furnaces, this one never reattained prewar production levels. And the community died, despite efforts to create a permanent town.

Climb away from Kirkman's Camp on an old roadbed and come to Point 13 at mile 6.2, very near the LBL boundary line. The Telegraph Trail veers left onto a narrower path and traverses a ridgeline. The ridgeline runs parallel to Bear Creek in rich woods with many carved beech trees. The path can be rocky in places.

Descend steeply to reach a flat and Point 14 beside Bear Creek. Cross the streambed beside some large trees and keep north along a line of trees to your right as the path traces a mown swath in a field broken by redbud trees. Soon, reach Fort Henry Road and the end of the trail. Ahead, across the road just beyond the picnic area, is the beginning of the North–South Trail.

ACCESS From the South Welcome Station, take FR 230, Fort Henry Road, 4.1 miles to FR 232. Turn right on FR 232 and follow it 0.1 mile, then keep forward as FR 232 turns to gravel 0.2 mile farther to dead-end at a turnaround. Look on the west side of the parking area for a trail signboard. Turn left at the signboard, following the red-blazed Telegraph Trail.

■ TELEGRAPH/PICKET TRAIL

TYPE Foot only   **DIFFICULTY** Easy   **LENGTH** 0.3 mile
USE Moderate   **CONDITION** Good
HIGHLIGHTS Connects Picket Loop Trail and Telegraph Trail
CONNECTIONS Telegraph Trail, Picket Loop Trail

THIS SHORT, FUNCTIONAL TRAIL is used to connect the Telegraph and Picket Loop Trails. The trail starts on the north side of Fort Henry Road at Point 26. From here, the blue-blazed Picket Loop Trail heads in both directions. Cross Fort Henry Road and head south, following the yellow blazes into an oak forest adjacent to a field. The singletrack footpath shortly comes alongside the field, then descends along a feeder stream of Fort Henry Branch. Step over a streambed draining the field below and reach Point 3 at 0.3 mile. From here, the Telegraph Trail leaves right 1.1 miles to end at Fort Henry trailhead and leaves left 0.2 mile to meet the Artillery Trail.

ACCESS From the South Welcome Station, take Forest Road 230, Fort Henry Road, 5.5 miles to the trailhead, at the top of a hill on your right. Look for a plastic sign on the right-hand side of the road with the number 26. This is Point 26 in the Fort Henry Trail System. Park on the left-hand side of the road. The yellow-blazed Telegraph/Picket Trail leaves south from the road.

■ TENNESSEE RIDGE TRAIL

TYPE Foot only   **DIFFICULTY** Easy   **LENGTH** 1.8 miles
USE Low   **CONDITION** Good   **HIGHLIGHTS** Solitude
CONNECTIONS Telegraph Trail, Peytona Trail

THIS TRAIL TRACES the physical divide between the watershed of the Cumberland River and the watershed of the Tennessee River. Called Tennessee Ridge, this North–South running rampart sheds water to the Tennessee on its west side and the Cumberland on its east side. A mostly level path, the trail undulates a bit as it passes a few clearings along its length. The Tennessee Ridge Trail can be used with the North–South Connector Trail, the Telegraph Trail, and the Peytona Trail to make an 8-mile loop.

Leave the junction with the Telegraph Trail, heading south. The blue-blazed Tennessee Ridge Trail passes by a former field growing up in pine, sumac, and young oaks. Sumac trees need full sunlight and often grow first in formerly cleared areas. The closed forest areas are primarily oaks. Over 20 species of oaks grow in Land Between The Lakes.

At 0.4 mile, the trail curves west, passing another former field on your right. Climb away from the field, reaching a high point at 0.8 mile. Descend briefly, then level off. Curve and undulate, as hollows drop off the ridgeline. The hollows to your left flow to Bear Creek, and the hollows to your right flow to Panther Creek. Obviously, some wild critters once roamed these parts. Nowadays, though, you are more likely to see wild turkeys and deer than panthers or bears.

Reach an area of pines and soon come to Point 16 and the end of the Tennessee Trail at mile 1.8. From here, the Peytona Trail leaves left 3.2 miles to meet the Telegraph Trail. The Peytona Trail leaves right 0.7 mile to meet the Artillery Trail.

ACCESS The Tennessee Ridge Trail is an interior trail. It can be reached by walking south from Fort Henry Road, Forest Road 230, on the North–South Connector Trail 0.8 mile to the Telegraph Trail, then 0.3 mile on the Telegraph Trail. You will be at the north end of the Tennessee Ridge Trail.

■ VOLUNTEER TRAIL

TYPE Foot only   **DIFFICULTY** Moderate   **LENGTH** 2.2 miles
USE Moderate to low   **CONDITION** Good
HIGHLIGHTS Three creeks, part of good loop
CONNECTIONS Piney Trail, Telegraph Trail

THE VOLUNTEER TRAIL is one of the more water-oriented trails at LBL. Its southward track alternately reaches creeks divided by low hills. The trail starts along Fort Henry Branch and heads south to meet North Fork Piney Creek. The path then spans an unnamed branch by wooden bridge, then makes a final dash for South Fork Piney Creek where it meets the Piney Trail. Technically, this trail can be accessed from Fort Henry Road; however, there is no parking along Fort Henry Road at the trail-head, which is off the road in the Fort Henry Branch bottom. I recommend using the first 0.4 mile of the Telegraph Trail to reach the Volunteer Trail. Turning east on the Piney Trail beyond the Volunteer Trail and returning via the Artillery and Telegraph Trails can make a quality 6.3-mile loop.

Start the Volunteer Trail by leaving Point 2 in the Fort Henry Trail System and heading south on the yellow-blazed path. Leave Fort Henry Branch bottom and climb amid some large hardwoods, topping out on a ridge at 0.5 mile. Turn left atop this ridge-line, now heading east. Much of the logging road is overgrown with spindly trees. North Fork Piney Creek Valley lies below you. Zigzag along the ridgeline, finally turning south on a finger ridge. Dive off the finger ridge to meet North Fork Piney Creek at 0.9 mile. Cross this streamshed and curve through a wide bottom to climb a low piney hill. Level off and climb a hickory-oak ridge. This time, turn west along the ridgeline and, as before, dive south to reach an unnamed stream at 1.6 miles. Span this feeder branch of South Fork Piney Creek via another wooden bridge and enter an attractive flat cloaked in cedar and maple. Pass a wildlife watering hole then ascend around a steep hill. Descend a final time, coming near a homesite on trail right, before you reach Point 21 at mile 2.2. Here, at South Fork Piney Creek, the Piney Trail leads left 1.0 mile to meet the Artillery Trail and leaves right to reach the Piney Campground entrance road after 1.3 miles.

ACCESS   From the South Welcome Station, take Forest Road 230, Fort Henry Road, 4.1 miles to FR 232. Keep on Fort Henry Road 0.3 mile farther, reaching a low spot in the road. A large culvert heads beneath the road here. Look left just past this culvert into the woods for the POINT 2 sign posted to a tree. Steps lead down from the road to this trail junction. The yellow-blazed Volunteer Trail heads south from here. Poor but usable parking for this trail is 0.1 mile back on the east side of Fort Henry Road over a small roadside culvert.

Nature Station Trails

THESE TRAILS EMANATE from the Nature Station, an environmental education area that offers animal viewing and interpretive information about LBL's wildlife, in addition to special programs. Nature Station trail maps can be obtained at both wel-come stations, Golden Pond Visitor Center and the Nature Station, as well as online.

■ CENTER FURNACE TRAIL

TYPE Foot only   **DIFFICULTY** Easy   **LENGTH** 0.3 mile
USE Moderate to heavy   **CONDITION** Good
HIGHLIGHTS Explores old iron furnace and surrounding lands with interpretive information
CONNECTIONS Hematite Trail

THIS INTERPRETIVE TRAIL gives a hands-on look at an old iron furnace, but also the land around it and the effects of iron working on this land. The community of Hematite, Kentucky, grew around the Center Furnace, one of eight iron furnaces that operated in what is now Land Between The Lakes.

Begin the Center Furnace Trail by climbing wide, wooden steps. Turn right and soon pass what was the general store of Hematite. Ahead is the cistern that stored runoff water from the general store's roof. Keep circling around a hill to reach one of the few old-growth trees in the immediate area. The furnace consumed an estimated 15–20 square miles of timber to operate while it was burning; this tree was spared for shade. Imagine that much of the surrounding forest denuded. Now, look and see how well the forest has recovered.

Center Furnace ruins

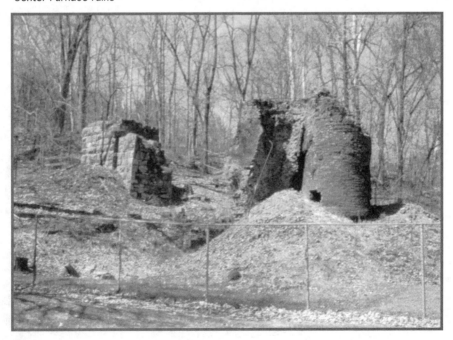

Ahead are the pits from which hematite, or iron ore, was dug. These pits still show obvious signs of man's hand on the landscape. Nearby is a replica of a charcoal pit, which demonstrates how charcoal used to fire the furnace was made from timber. The charcoal makers, known as colliers, had to be meticulous in the construction and lighting of these charcoal pits. If the fires got too hot, less charcoal would result or, worse, the pit would explode.

Come to the hill overlooking the furnace ruins. Brick and rock were used in building this furnace, which is surrounded by a fence. Ahead is a monument to one of the idea men behind the furnace.

Today's iron production is much more eco-friendly. Center Furnace is but a reminder of the advances in iron production that we use today.

ACCESS   From the entrance of Golden Pond Visitor Center, take Woodlands Trace 9.4 miles north to Silver Trail Road, Forest Road 133. Turn right on Silver Trail Road and follow it 3.0 miles to the Center Furnace trailhead, on your right.

■ HEMATITE TRAIL

TYPE Foot only   **DIFFICULTY** Easy   **LENGTH** 2.2 miles
USE Moderate to heavy   **CONDITION** Good
HIGHLIGHTS Wildlife viewing, boardwalk, photo blind, big trees
CONNECTIONS Center Furnace Trail, Long Creek Trail

THIS WALK ALONG THE HEMATITE TRAIL, which passes along Hematite Lake, is worth every step. The lake itself is an impoundment of Long Creek. Hematite is the ore, primarily iron, that was found in the area. The abundance of hematite led to the building of an iron furnace, Center Furnace, nearby. A community, aptly named Hematite, developed around the activity of Center Furnace. In the first half of the 1800s, "ol' Kentuck'" was one of the leading iron producers in a young United States.

But the iron era came and went. Fast-forward to the 1960s, when the Tennessee Valley Authority dammed Long Creek in this valley. Wildlife soon discovered this watery refuge and wetland. Now, you can enjoy this mostly level loop trail and maybe see some of that wildlife for yourself.

The Hematite Trail starts from the upper end of the Hematite Picnic Area. Follow the gravel road leading past the two-tiered outflow of the Hematite Lake dam. The trail remains wide along the right-hand bank of 90-acre Hematite Lake. The dam is to your left. At 0.1 mile, the trail narrows and begins to meander along the south-facing

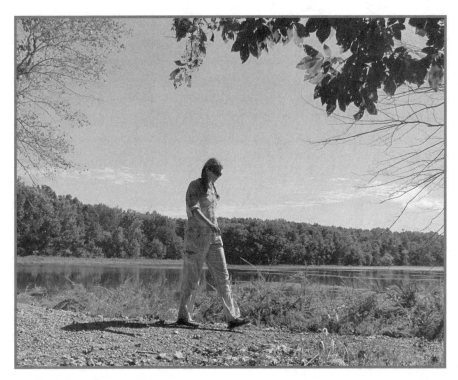

Hiking the Hematite Lake Trail

shoreline of Hematite Lake. The shallow lake has abundant growth on its surface. Pass a few short but wide boardwalks spanning intermittent streams.

Work uphill around an old rock quarry where limestone was dug. Added to the iron ore, limestone helped raise the temperature of the ore and aided in ridding impurities from the iron. Return to the lakeside, reaching a bluff with a view at 0.3 mile. Turtles will be sunning on logs. Occasional stands of river cane obscure the view of Hematite Lake.

Turn away from the lake, working around a low point that is subject to flooding. The trail returns to the lake, reaching a boardwalk at 0.8 mile. This wetland can look vastly different season to season. You are likely to see beaver dams here. Three elevated bridges span streams on this upper end of Hematite Lake. The last bridge crosses Long Creek. Just after Long Creek, a side trail leads left to a peninsula and contemplation bench overlooking the impoundment. Look for raccoon tracks on the boardwalk.

Return to the main boardwalk, which passes large bottomland hardwoods, such as tulip trees. The boardwalk ends on the south shore of Hematite Lake. Begin heading east, undulating between small streamlets spanned by boardwalks. At mile 1.3, a side trail leads left to the lake and another boardwalk.

Cruise along the shoreline over low hills that offer occasional lake vistas. Swing around one last arm of the lake to reach the dam. Look for bank anglers trying their luck from the dam. A set of concrete steps leads across the outflow of the dam. Beyond the steps, turn right and complete the loop.

ACCESS From the entrance of Golden Pond Visitor Center, head north on Woodlands Trace for 7.0 miles to Mulberry Flats Road, Forest Road 135. Turn right on Mulberry Flats Road and follow it 4.0 miles to FR 134. Turn left on FR 134 and follow it a mile to Hematite Lake Picnic Area, on your left just before Center Furnace ruins. The Hematite Lake Trail starts in the back of the picnic area.

■ HONKER TRAIL

TYPE Foot only   **DIFFICULTY** Easy   **LENGTH** 4.5 miles
USE Moderate to heavy   **CONDITION** Good
HIGHLIGHTS Varied ecosystems, lake views, wildlife
CONNECTIONS Woodland Walk

THIS IS THE longest loop of the Nature Station Trails. The trail circles Honker Lake, making for a great day hike. Along the way, it passes through lakeside wetlands, hardwood forest, open lands, and shoreline. The hills aren't too steep or long, making it hikeable by most everyone, despite being 4.5 miles long.

Leave the Honker Lake access road and begin walking south, away from the Nature Station, on a raised trail bed. Come alongside Long Creek. Bridge Long Creek and begin circling around Honker Lake in attractive woodland. Shortly, cross two smaller streambeds by bridge. The Honker Trail climbs a low hill, crosses another small bridge, then dips to flatland again. Curve past a piled ramp left over from the iron-ore days. It is likely that this ramp was used to load iron ore from nearby pits onto sturdy wagons for transport to Center Furnace.

Pass under a power line at 1.2 miles. Turn away from the lake, picking up a roadbed for a minute, then leave left, passing an old iron-ore pit filled with water, frogs, salamanders, and other aquatic wildlife. Ahead, the trail turns left, but a spur path leads right to a second ore pit.

The Honker Trail returns to a bluff overlooking the lake and cruises to meet Forest Road 138, just past a trail map signboard. Lake Barkley is across from the forest road. Turn left and head toward Honker Dam. Pass around the metal gate at mile 2.1 and cross the long, low dam, which offers extensive lake views. You will likely run into people fishing here.

Climb over a hill at the end of the dam. The woods atop the hill contrast with the open lake area. Dip to cross the dam outflow via a concrete path. To your left are the Goose Islands. Honker Lake is a winter wildlife refuge. Trace a piney peninsula, and shortly begin circling around the lake again. Pass beneath a power line at mile 3.0. The Honker Trail then bridges a spring branch to climb an oak-hickory hill. Pick up a roadbed and descend back to bottomland. Slice through the bottomland via a raised trail bed.

The Honker Trail opens to a field. The Nature Station is atop the hill ahead. Meet the Woodland Walk at mile 4.0 and veer left, sharing the trail bed with the shorter trail as it curves around a peninsula, then reaches a small cemetery. Pass by a limestone pit, used to build the furnace and to melt the ore into iron. Reach a trail junction. The Honker Trail leaves left and heads just a few feet to complete its loop.

ACCESS   From the entrance of Golden Pond Visitor Center, take Woodlands Trace 7 miles north to Mulberry Flat Road, FR 135. Turn right on Mulberry Flat Road and follow it 4 miles to FR 134. Turn left on FR 134 and follow it 1 mile to the right turn, just across from the Center Furnace. Follow this access road a short distance past the Long Creek trailhead to the Honker Trail parking area, on your right.

■ LONG CREEK TRAIL

TYPE All access   **DIFFICULTY** Easy   **LENGTH** 0.4 mile
USE Moderate to heavy   **CONDITION** Good
HIGHLIGHTS Wheelchair-accessible path
CONNECTIONS None

THIS ALL-ACCESS TRAIL leaves from near Center Furnace and leads through bottomland of Long Creek as it flows between Hematite and Honker Lakes. Big sycamore trees reach overhead. The miniloop at the end of the trail offers angling possibilities.

This federally designated national recreation trail heads away from the parking area toward Long Creek and enters a bottomland dominated by sycamores. Notice how the entire trailway has been elevated above the forest, the vines, and the river cane. Ahead, a side trail leads left to a dead end. The loop portion of the trail makes a small circle. The path comes directly alongside Long Creek before making its turn.

Long Creek forms a loop here, too, but the creek takes a much longer distance to circle back around than does the trail.

Long Creek makes its turn and you are soon along the creek again. If you see chicken wire around some trees, be aware that it is to keep beavers from chewing the trees down. Beavers have made a major comeback at LBL and often their hard work is unwanted. The Long Creek Trail completes its miniloop at 0.2 mile. Backtrack to the trailhead.

ACCESS   From the entrance of Golden Pond Visitor Center, take Woodlands Trace 7.0 miles north to Mulberry Flat Road, FR 135. Turn right on Mulberry Flat Road and follow it 4.0 miles to FR 134. Turn left on FR 134 and follow it a mile to the right turn into the Long Creek trailhead parking area, just across from the Center Furnace ruins.

■ NATURE STATION CONNECTOR TRAIL

TYPE Foot only   DIFFICULTY Moderate   LENGTH 4.8 miles
USE Moderate   CONDITION Good
HIGHLIGHTS Connects North–South Trail to Nature Station, attractive creeks
CONNECTIONS North–South Trail, Token Trail Spring Spur Trail, Woodland Walk, Honker Trail

THE NATURE STATION TRAILHEAD is an alternative starting spot for hiking the North–South Trail via the Nature Station Connector Trail. However, the Nature Station Connector Trail makes a good hike on its own. It leaves the Nature Station, crosses a stream, ascends a west-leading ridgeline, and then drops into Racetrack Hollow, crossing Fulton Creek. It then ascends back onto the ridgeline to intersect Token Trail Spring Spur Trail and Silver Trail Road. The spur trail descends to a spring and campsite in upper Racetrack Hollow. The Nature Station Connector Trail then traces Silver Trail Road to cross Woodlands Trace. The path dips into the Tennessee River drainage here. It works down to Duncan Creek, passing through an attractive wooded flat, crossing Duncan Creek and several feeder branches before intersecting the North–South Trail beside a large field.

Leave the Nature Station trailhead and follow the mown path right, soon reaching a gravel road. Turn left on the gravel road and descend to reach a trail sign. Veer left here, following the arrow that states "North–South Trail." Pass by a tall, two-trunked sycamore and continue around a field. Drop to a stream called Negro Row Branch. Many African Americans, most likely slaves, worked at the nearby Center Iron Furnace and lived along this stream. The thick woods belie any indication of settlement. However, look down at the gravel road below you. The strange blue rocks are slag. Slag rocks are the cooled impurities left over from the iron-making process. Ironworkers recycled this slag by using it for roads.

Cross Negro Row Branch via culvert and ascend, reaching a metal gate at 0.6 mile. Turn left here; the yellow blazes head west on Forest Road 314. Soon, pass a wildlife pond among the hickory-oak woods. Pines are scattered on the ridge too. At mile 1.3, FR 312 leads right. Keep forward on FR 314. At mile 1.6, the Nature Station Connector Trail splits right, off the forest road. The canopy closes in overhead, except for a couple of small clearings. Curve into Racetrack Hollow, crossing Fulton Creek at 2.2 miles. This flat offers potential camping, especially if Fulton Creek is flowing.

Legend has it that Racetrack Hollow got its name back during the Prohibition era, when moonshine making was big here. Moonshine runners would practice their elusive driving techniques in the hollow on their "corn likker" runs from Between The Rivers, as Land Between The Lakes was then known, to the big cities.

The Nature Station Connector Trail ascends away from Racetrack Hollow into a young forest atop a ridge. Follow this spine through a wildlife clearing at mile 2.5. The going is easy for the next half mile. At 3.0 miles, intersect the Token Trail Spring Spur Trail. It leaves right a half mile to reach Token Trail spring and campsite. The Nature Station Connector Trail keeps forward, passing around a metal gate. Turn right on paved Silver Trail Road and follow it 0.3 mile to reach Woodlands Trace. Cross Woodlands Trace, following the yellow blazes into woodland. The Nature Station Connector Trail shortly dips off the hickory-oak ridge and into the upper reaches of Duncan Creek. Step over a couple of streambeds. The hollow widens, but the trail stays in the hills north of Duncan Creek. An old homesite lies to the left of the trail near a pine grove. Look here for metal relics.

At mile 4.0, reach a flat and cross Duncan Creek. Keep downstream and enter a hardwood and cedar grove. The trail turns away from Duncan Creek, climbing a small hill, then descends to a feeder branch before reaching a fast-disappearing clearing on a second hill. Drop to another feeder branch that is shaded by some big trees. A large field is visible to the right. Skirt the margin between the creek to your left and the field to your right, spanning the unnamed stream on a wooden bridge. Pass under a power line and shortly intersect the North–South Trail at mile 4.8. Notice the big tulip trees near the junction. From here, the North–South Trail leaves right toward North Welcome Station. It leaves left toward Golden Pond.

ACCESS From the entrance of Golden Pond Visitor Center, take Woodlands Trace 9.4 miles north to Silver Trail Road, FR 133. Turn right on Silver Trail Road and follow it 3.0 miles to the Nature Station trailhead on your left near the picnic pavilion, before reaching the main Nature Station parking area.

■ TOKEN TRAIL SPRING SPUR TRAIL

TYPE Foot only   **DIFFICULTY** Easy   **LENGTH** 0.5 mile   **USE** Low to moderate

CONDITION Good   **HIGHLIGHTS** Campsite and spring in wooded hollow

CONNECTIONS Nature Station Connector Trail

THIS PATH DESCENDS from Silver Trail Road and the Nature Station Connector Trail to the upper end of Racetrack Hollow. Backpackers needing a quick campsite use this trail, as do backpackers leaving from the Nature Station trailhead.

The yellow-blazed Token Trail Spring Spur Trail begins where the Nature Station Connector Trail meets Silver Trail Road. Follow the yellow rectangles off of the ridgeline. Descend along a feeder branch of Fulton Creek. Reach a flat where several streambeds converge at 0.2 mile. This is the upper end of Racetrack Hollow.

The trail turns east down Racetrack Hollow. Tall trees shade the forest floor. The trail crosses over a streamlet coming in from the right. Reach a flat and campsite just beyond this streamlet. Here, the yellow-blazed trail turns up the streamlet and shortly reaches Token Trail Spring. This spring emerges from the hillside and forms a shallow pool. Another small campsite is at the spring.

Token Trail Spring gets its name from the nearby iron-producing Center Furnace. In the mid-1800s, workers at Center Furnace were paid in silver. The company wagon brought this silver down the road that became known as Silver Trail Road. After the Civil War, and the end of cost-saving slave labor, Center Furnace limped along, until other factors such as depletion of nearby timber to fire the furnace and newer iron-producing technology shut the furnace down.

In the early 1900s, the fires at Center Furnace were started again. This time the employees were not paid in silver, but in tokens. These tokens were redeemable only at the company store. The Silver Trail then became the Token Trail. Finally, in 1912, Center Furnace cooled for the last time.

ACCESS From the entrance of Golden Pond Visitor Center, take Woodlands Trace 9.4 miles north to Silver Trail Road, Forest Road 133. Turn right on Silver Trail Road and follow it 0.3 mile to a gated gravel road on your left. The yellow-blazed spur trail leaves left just beyond the gate. Do not block the gate when parking.

■ WOODLAND WALK

TYPE Foot only   **DIFFICULTY** Easy   **LENGTH** 1.0 mile   **USE** Moderate to heavy

CONDITION Good   **HIGHLIGHTS** Lake views, big trees, old cemetery, limestone quarry

CONNECTIONS Honker Trail

THIS TRAIL IS a good leg stretcher for Nature Station visitors, since it departs from the Nature Station parking area. This trail was named for the Kentucky Woodlands National Wildlife Refuge, which was along the Cumberland River before Lake Barkley and Land Between The Lakes came to be. The refuge was established in 1935 and covered 65,000 acres. The refuge focused on protecting and increasing waterfowl populations. To this day, the lakes around the Nature Station harbor many waterfowl during winter.

You may see some waterfowl on Honker Lake from this trail. However, the Hematite and Honker Trails are better for overall waterfowl viewing. Start the Woodland Walk by leaving north from the Nature Station, left as you face it. The Woodland Walk descends past an overlook and down many wood steps to a field. You may see fallow deer in the field below. Walk the margin between field and wood, entering the forest to the right.

Walk along a north-facing slope. Notice the moisture-loving trees, such as wild cherry, sycamore, and sugar maple. Shortly, join the Honker Trail. The two paths then circle around a picnic area on a peninsula. The Honker Lake canoe rental area, open during summer, stands along the shore to the left. The Woodland Walk cruises

LBL historic graveyard

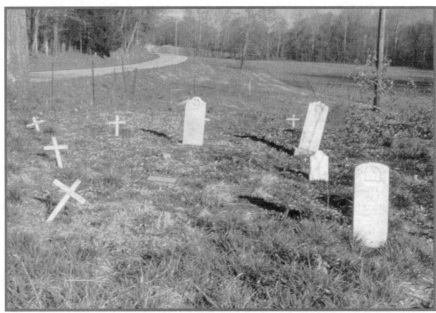

beneath tall pines. These loblolly and shortleaf pines were planted in the 1930s to check erosion and provide food for wildlife.

Circle around the peninsula, passing more contemplation and observation benches. Look for a large multitrunked cherry tree to the left of the trail, then come to a small, unnamed cemetery. In the late 1990s, some former LBL residents formed a group called Rescue Our Cemeteries. They have found over 200 graveyards in LBL. Not much is known about this unnamed cemetery, but a Chinese cemetery is nearby. There, Chinese laborers who worked at Center Furnace, along with other workers and possibly slaves, are interred. The Chinese cemetery is directly behind the Nature Station on the inside perimeter of the Woodland Walk.

The Woodland Walk keeps forward past the small, unmarked cemetery. Ahead, the path reaches a junction. The Honker Trail leaves left here, and the Woodland Trail curves right, past a limestone quarry. Limestone was used to build the iron furnace and was used in the iron blasting process. The Woodland Walk curves up a hill and shortly arrives at the south side of the Nature Station parking area.

ACCESS   From the entrance of Golden Pond Visitor Center, head north on Woodlands Trace 9.2 miles to Silver Trail Road, Forest Road 133. Turn right on Silver Trail Road and follow it 3.1 miles to dead-end at the Woodlands Nature Station. The Woodland Walk leaves from the north side of the parking area, to the left as you face the Nature Station.

North–South Trail

THE NORTH–SOUTH TRAIL is LBL's master path. This federally designated National Recreation Trail runs the entire length of the LBL peninsula—60 miles—from near Dover in Tennessee to near Grand Rivers in Kentucky. Along the way it traverses many different environments, including oak-covered ridges, lush bottomland, and rolling lakeshore.

The North–South Trail begins at the South Welcome Station. Here, it leaves Bear Creek Valley and ascends the Tennessee Divide. To the west, streams drain into the Tennessee River. To the east, streams drain into the Cumberland River. The trail runs through grand forests of oak and hickory broken by sporadic wildlife clearings—meadows that offer a contrast to the rich woodland. Spur trails lead to springs and campsites, and one of five trail shelters, giving backpackers a place to overnight.

As the North–South Trail continues north, it leaves the ridgeline, dipping into the Laura Furnace Fork watershed. Equestrians also enjoy the North–South Trail for a 10-mile stretch here. The trail then dips into Turkey Creek, just one of many bottomlands where sycamore and other moisture-loving trees grow thick and tall over spring wildflowers. Fields break some valley bottoms. The fields offer extended vistas and food for wildlife. Trail travelers will notice old cemeteries from the days when the peninsula was settled. A discerning eye will also spot evidence of homesites, from squared-off foundation stones to leftover wire fence.

The North–South Trail comes very near Golden Pond Visitor Center around the midpoint. Hikers and mountain bikers share the trail beyond the visitor center. The path dips west toward Kentucky Lake and begins a pattern of reaching into richly wooded hollows. You'll then span winding streams that pass through thick valley bottoms, passing beside Kentucky Lake, only to rise and traverse stately oak ridges. The trail descends from the ridgetops and reaches the lake again, where far-reaching vistas across the water await. A variety of campsites, springs, and shelters are situated along the trail here. Finally, the North–South Trail swings alongside tall bluffs overlooking Kentucky Lake. Steep hollows break these bluffs and make for a challenging and scenic ending to one of America's better long trails.

Iron Mountain Trail Shelter

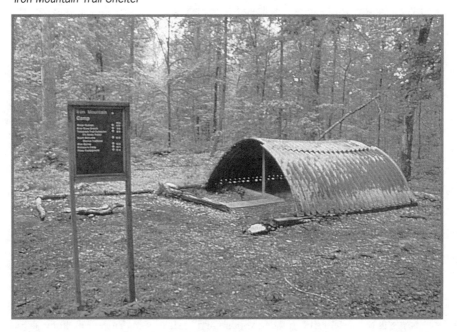

Multiuse is a great aspect of this path—hikers, mountain bikers, and equestrians all get a taste of the North–South Trail. Many folks backpack the trail in its entirety. Others hike it section by section, and some use it as part of loop hikes, or in the case of the north half of the trail, for mountain biking rides and loops.

Trail treaders should note that use of the North–South Trail is seasonal. The best time to backpack this path is from mid-September to the end of May, though equestrians and mountain bikers tend to use it during summer. Heat, overgrown vegetation, and ticks will make backpackers miserable during the warm season. By the way, consider using lightweight gaiters for added tick protection. Most LBL visitors focus on water-oriented activities from June to September.

As the barren trees open the woods, winter offers the most solitude and surprisingly frequent wildlife viewings. The five shelters along the trail offer refuge from the wind and elements. As life renews itself in spring, trail trekking can be excellent. The days are lengthening, many streams have water flowing—adding more camping opportunities—and the ticks are few in number. Also, the wildflowers are blooming—LBL has flowering plants that rival many more famous trail destinations. As the trees leaf out, the trail is still worth a visit, especially for mountain bikers—since warmth dries out the path. In summer, limit your hikes to morning and evening. It is time again to hit the trail after the first cold fronts blow through in September.

Many believe that fall reveals LBL at its best. The trails are dry, the bugs are limited, and autumn colors are putting on a show. The only downside: water. Water can be limited to springs only, so you may have to walk a bit extra on spur trails to quench your thirst. All North–South Spur Trails are detailed following the North–South Trail description.

The following North–South Trail description is broken into four segments, heading from south to north. This is the best way to travel for two reasons: it keeps the sun at your back and keeps with the spirit of the granddaddy long trail, the Appalachian Trail, which is primarily hiked south to north. These segments can be covered by overnight backpack or by day hiking, though day hikers may have to consult an LBL road map to place their automobile if they want to break each segment into small sections. Consult the North–South Trail Log at the end of the trail description to help you plan your hikes. Backpackers leaving their autos at either the North Welcome Station or the South Welcome Station are encouraged to register their cars before leaving on a trip.

■ NORTH–SOUTH TRAIL:
South Welcome to Ginger Creek Road

LENGTH 13.7 miles   **CONDITION** Excellent
HIGHS Wildlife viewing, Iron Mountain fire tower and trail shelter
LOWS Limited water and camping   **DIFFICULTY** Moderate
TIPS Plan your water carefully during this section

AFTER LEAVING THE SOUTH WELCOME STATION, the trail ascends to the Tennessee Divide and faithfully follows it to Ginger Creek Road. The path does some snaking among the watersheds of the Tennessee and Cumberland rivers, but it manages to keep north, often on two-track jeep trails used to access the numerous wildlife clearings atop the ridgeline. Camping opportunities are limited, and you must plan to hike at least 8.0 miles to Brier Rose Branch if you want to overnight near water. If time constraints force a shorter first day, consider taking the Telegraph Trail (Bear Creek Loop), south from the welcome station, then camping at Kirkman's Camp the first night, 1.6 miles in. The next day, backpackers can keep west on the Telegraph Trail to intersect the Fort Henry North–South Trail Connector then rejoin the North–South Trail.

Fill your water bottle before you start, as it is several miles before trailside water is available. The North–South Trail starts inauspiciously, leaving the picnic area near South Welcome Station as a narrow footpath blazed in white. Angle up the slope of a hill. Woodlands Trace is to your right. Pass through rich forest scattered with beech trees. Join a ridgeline and follow it generally uphill, topping out on a knob, before descending to reach a roadbed at mile 1.0. The North–South Trail turns left, following the roadbed past a field and pond to the left.

Wind along the ridge past numerous pine stands, eventually coming to a small hilltop field. Pass alongside, then through, a small field before reaching a junction at mile 2.0. Here, the Fort Henry North–South Trail Connector leaves left 1.4 miles to intersect the Telegraph Trail.

The North–South Trail keeps northwest. It now joins the Tennessee Divide. To the west, Panther Creek flows into the Tennessee River. To the east, Brandon Springs Branch flows into the Cumberland River. Soon, pass the first of numerous wildlife clearings. At the second clearing past the junction, look right, into the woods, for a circular wire fence. This is a well from an old homesite. The forest service found and fenced these wells to keep unsuspecting woods trompers from falling in.

The trail keeps between 500 and 600 feet in elevation, working along old doubletrack jeep roads among an oak-hickory forest. At mile 2.8, it leaves right as a singletrack path, only to join another wildlife access road, thus avoiding a meadow atop a hill. The canopy gives way in spots. At mile 3.9, a road splits left to a clearing. Keep right here, as indicated by a sign with an arrow. Shortly, pass a long, prominent field on your right. Make a solid incline at mile 4.7, topping out near a meadow. Circle around the right-hand side of the meadow. At mile 5.1, reach a pine plantation, then work down to a road split in a gap at mile 5.3. Keep left, staying on mostly level ground. At mile 6.0, watch for the North–South Trail leaving left, away from the more used road heading into another pine plantation. This area becomes confusing. Shortly, reach another junction, where a sign marks the area as 8 N 1. Turn right, as indicated by signage. Split left at the next junction, mile 6.3, on a rutted gravel track flanked by young shortleaf pines.

Resume a more followable trail segment that leads to the Morgan Cemetery at mile 6.9. Join gravel Forest Road 222, passing more wildlife clearings. At mile 7.5, just before reaching FR 221, the North–South Trail veers right into the woods, making a singletrack beneath pines. Intersect the Brier Rose Branch Spur Trail at mile 7.9. Here, the spur trail leads right 0.2 mile to a spring and campsite. Turn away from the spur trail, running alongside a field to your left to cross FR 221 at mile 8.1. Join a wildlife access doubletrack, resuming the ridgeline. Sassafras is a prominent understory species here.

Sassafras was one of America's first exports. Colonists thought the aromatic roots were a cure-all. The oil was used to perfume soap, and roots were used to make sassafras tea. Look for a small tree or shrub with mitten-shaped leaves, though the leaves can vary. Sassafras ranges from Maine southwest to Florida to Texas.

Pass beside a very attractive meadow dotted with pine trees. At mile 9.0, look left for a side trail leading to the small Fuqua Cemetery atop a hill. Keep in a mix of pine and some hardwoods. At mile 9.4, look for a foot-high concrete marker beside the trail. It is a U.S. Geological Survey marker from 1934. Leave the pine grove, resuming the natural hickory-oak forest composition. Interestingly, only 3% of LBL is forested in pine, and half of that is planted pine. Most of the native pine is shortleaf.

Pass more fields amid the woods before climbing to reach Iron Mountain Camp at mile 10.9. This is the first of five trail shelters. These open-fronted shelters are curved steel structures. They have a wall on the back and a gravel floor. They have room for four backpackers and their gear. Water is available at a spigot on the building near the Iron Mountain fire tower, just up the hill from the shelter. Hikers can climb the fire tower at their own risk during daylight hours only. Built in 1955, this tower and facility is maintained by the Tennessee Division of Forestry. A railroad tie manufacturing company, Well Heath, leased this land to the state of Tennessee for 99 years. All land around this lease is federally owned. The lease expires in 2054.

The North–South Trail circles around the tower area on a singletrack path to reach paved FR 211, Fire Tower Road. Cross the road to reenter woods on a single-track path. Circle around a large wildlife clearing to your left. Stay below the field in this attractive, hilly area. Pass a second clearing and keep north, reaching a piney area atop a hill. Keep forward, passing one last clearing before reaching Ginger Creek Road, FR 205, at mile 13.7 and the end of this section.

ACCESS *South Welcome Trailhead:* From Dover, TN, head south on US 79 5.0 miles to access Woodlands Trace. Turn right on Woodlands Trace and drive north 3.4 miles to reach the South Welcome Station on your right. Park at the welcome station. However, the North–South Trail begins at the picnic area northwest of the welcome station across Woodlands Trace and Fort Henry Road.

Ginger Creek Road Trailhead: From the South Welcome station, head north on Woodlands Trace 9.7 miles to gravel FR 205, Ginger Creek Road. FR 205 is the first left turn after the Great Western Iron Furnace. Follow FR 205 0.9 mile to reach the crest of the Tennessee Divide. Look for the signage marking the North–South Trail. There is ample parking for three to four cars at the trail crossing.

■ NORTH–SOUTH TRAIL:
Ginger Creek Road to Golden Pond

LENGTH 15.1 miles   **CONDITION** Fair to good, can be very bad in spots
HIGHS Creeks, homesites, many camping opportunities
LOWS Potentially rutted and muddy trail   **DIFFICULTY** Moderate
TIPS Slip off to the low side of the trail when encountering horses

THIS TRAIL SECTION has some ups and downs, both literally and figuratively. Leaving Ginger Creek Road, the North–South Trail keeps along the Tennessee Divide then crosses Woodlands Trace, undulating among the hollows of Laura Furnace Creek. Horses begin using the trail where Wranglers Trail 8 runs in conjunction with the North–South Trail. Unfortunately, sections of the path have become rutted and sometimes muddy from the equestrian traffic. However, hold no grudge against these riders, as 10 miles of the path are designated for both horse and foot traffic. Besides, most equestrians greet you with a smile as they enjoy the LBL in their own way.

After leaving the Laura Furnace Fork watershed, the North–South Trail resumes the ridgeline, intersecting the Central Hardwoods Scenic Trail before reaching the Golden Pond Spur Trail. The spur path leads a short distance to Golden Pond trailhead and the end of this segment. Backpackers will enjoy this trail segment, as it offers numerous springs and camping opportunities all along the route, including trail shelters and spur trails to view bison from near their camp.

Start this trail segment by leaving north from Forest Road 205, Ginger Creek Road. Climb a hill and undulate along a doubletrack path to reach a trail junction at 0.2 mile. Here, the Model Loop Trail leads right 0.8 mile to Bison Hideaway campsite. This site lies in a hollow just outside the fenced Bison Range, where you can glimpse the large shaggy creatures. Hikers can continue along the Bison Range on the Model Loop Trail to rejoin the North–South Trail after 2.5 more miles. The North–South Trail keeps forward, then veers left, tracing a level track near a wildlife clearing with a watering hole beside the path. Reenter woods, then drop off the ridgeline. Curve downhill to reach a trail junction at mile 1.5. A yellow-blazed spur trail leads left for 75 yards to Prospector's Place campsite and spring. A home once stood here and relics such as washtubs remain.

The North–South Trail courses over a streambed and inclines to regain the ridgecrest. Shortly, pass some wildlife clearings, then, at mile 2.5, pass a wildlife clearing with a silting pond on your right. Split a final, large, narrow ridgetop field before reaching the north end of the Model Loop Trail at mile 3.1. It leaves right 1.5 miles to reach the Homeplace trailhead.

Soon the North–South Trail veers left and crosses Woodlands Trace. Here begins the 10-mile section of the North–South Trail, which is open to horses. Undulate along the ridgeline near Woodlands Trace, briefly picking up FR 356 at mile 3.7. Wranglers Trail 8 now runs in conjunction with the North–South Trail. Descend to a gullied streambed in the Laura Furnace Creek watershed to cross the Kentucky state line at mile 4.0. Yellow blazes painted on trees mark the state line. Pass the Rushing Family Cemetery at mile 4.5. The graves range from rough fieldstones to marked tombs. Turn left to cross Laura Furnace Creek. Broken and overgrown fields shield relics of homes once in this valley. Pass along a bluffline overlooking a feeder branch of Laura Furnace Creek. Wranglers Trail 8 and the North–South Trail briefly separate along an old lane. Here, the North–South Trail crosses a streambed via wooden bridge, the first bridge of the entire trail. At mile 5.0, the North–South Trail, now reunited with the bridle path, crosses FR 165.

Ascend away from FR 165, passing the tiny Blossey Cemetery. Drop to step over a feeder branch of Laura Furnace Creek in a rocky area. The North–South Trail then picks up the access road to Bullock Cemetery. Walk a few feet on the access road then intersect the Walker Line Trail at mile 6.1. The Walker Line Trail leaves left, going

2.8 miles to Rushing Creek Campground. The campground has potable water, hot showers, and lakeside camping for a fee.

Descend away from the junction to another feeder branch of Laura Furnace Creek. Climb out of the small valley to reach a pine thicket and FR 406 at mile 7.2. Here, Wranglers Trail 8 leaves right, while the North–South Trail keeps forward along a narrower track. Come near Woodlands Trace, then reach bottomland, now in West Fork Laura Furnace Creek drainage. Ascend again, pass by a pine grove, and make one last dip before reaching a trail junction at mile 8.8. Here, the Mountain Laurel Spring Spur Trail leaves left 0.8 mile to a reliable spring and backcountry campsite in upper Redd Hollow.

The North–South Trail comes to a confusing area in a gap at mile 9.0. Old roadbeds spur off in all directions. Look for the arrow on a sign leading forward and slightly left. Two paths run parallel but soon come together, then make a sharp final drop to reach West Fork Laura Furnace Creek at mile 9.4. Here, the Laura Furnace Fork Spur Trail leads right 0.8 mile to the Laura Furnace Fork trail shelter and spring. The spur trail then continues for 0.8 mile to reach Fords Bay Road, FR 170.

West Fork flows longer than many streams in LBL. Keep forward and cross West Fork, then reach a bluff overlooking the streambed. Climb to make Fords Bay Road, FR 170, at mile 10.4. Here, yellow blazes lead right to the Laura Furnace Fork Spur Trail, then 2.7 miles farther to Wranglers Campground via forest roads and horse trails. Camping, showers, a small store, and a telephone are all at Wranglers Campground.

The North–South Trail descends from the road into the Turkey Creek watershed. Cross a streambed that is usually flowing from a spring just above the trail crossing, then reach the unsigned Colson Overlook Spur Trail at mile 10.9. This spur leads uphill to a picnic area and overlook of Kentucky Lake far to the west. The North–South Trail continues forward as the field remains to your right. Make bottomland, crossing Turkey Creek then a feeder branch before reaching another trail junction at mile 11.5. Here, the Turkey Spring/School House Hollow Spring Spur Trail leaves left 0.3 mile to School House Hollow Spring and 0.3 mile farther to Turkey Spring and campsite.

The North–South Trail ascends from the junction, gaining a gravelly, oak ridge broken by a wildlife clearing. Keep below a large clearing to your right, where a horse trail runs along the field. At mile 12.7, pass behind the Compton Cemetery, then join FR 342. The North–South Trail now runs in conjunction with Wranglers Trail 11. At mile 13.5, leave FR 342. This marks the end of the joint trail use with equestrians, as Wranglers Trail 11 leaves right. Climb a hill to pass under a power line and reach the Ross Cemetery, with its many small stone markers.

Follow a singletrack path through old woods with a young forest in the distance to your right. Come near a large building at the LBL maintenance shop. Curve around a hollow and pass through a stand of locust to emerge near Woodlands Trace and an RV dump station at mile 14.5. Potable water from a water pump is available here. Cross Woodlands Trace and look for signs indicating the North–South Trail. Parallel Woodlands Trace and dip to a streambed spanned by a bridge, then climb to reach a trail junction at mile 14.9. Here, the Golden Pond Spur Trail leads right 0.2 mile to the Golden Pond trailhead and the end of this trail section. The Central Hardwoods Scenic Trail leads left toward Fenton and right a short distance to the Golden Pond Visitor Center. From here, it is 31.2 miles north to the North Welcome Station. The Golden Pond trailhead marks the point where bicyclers can also enjoy the North–South Trail.

ACCESS *Ginger Creek Road Trailhead:* From the South Welcome Station, head north on Woodlands Trace 9.7 miles to gravel FR 205, Ginger Creek Road. FR 205 is the first left turn after the Great Western Iron Furnace. Follow FR 205 0.9 mile to reach the crest of the Tennessee Divide. Look for the signs marking the North–South Trail. There is ample parking for three to four cars at the trail crossing.

Golden Pond Trailhead: Golden Pond Visitor Center is centrally located at LBL. It can be reached from the east on I-24 at Exit 65 via US 68/KY 80, from the north on I-24 from Exit 31 via KY 453 South, from the west by KY 80, and from the south by US 79 and Woodlands Trace. The Golden Pond trailhead is located on Golden Pond Road, the short road that connects Woodlands Trace to US 68/KY 80, just south of the Golden Pond Visitor Center. Look for the gravel parking area beside a few covered snack and drink machines.

■ NORTH–SOUTH TRAIL: Golden Pond to Duncan Bay

LENGTH 18.0 miles   **CONDITION** Very good
HIGHS Vistas of Kentucky Lake, lakeshore camping, bridges over creeks for mountain bikes
LOWS Most hills of any segment   **DIFFICULTY** Moderate to difficult, due to length of segment and hills   **TIPS** Hikers and mountain bikers share the trail

THIS TRAIL SECTION is very scenic and offers a variety of environments, including hickory-oak ridges that break up the lush bottomlands. Here begins the trail portion that passes along the scenic bays of Kentucky Lake, offering a watery contrast of massive proportions, especially after traveling amid LBL's thick woodlands. You will probably see and undoubtedly hear the low hum of tugboats pushing barges up and down Kentucky Lake, as they ply the Tennessee River with their loads. Camping options increase with the lakeside trail segments, along with trail shelters and springs. Trail travelers will also notice the numerous bridges that span most creeks of any size. These were installed to make the North–South Trail more mountain bike friendly, as pedalers also use the trail from Golden Pond north all the way to the North Welcome Station.

Start by taking the short Golden Pond Spur Trail to cross Woodlands Trace and reach the North–South Trail. Turn right on the North–South Trail, heading north on a singletrack footpath, dipping to cross a small streambed. Climb a steep hillside where many blueberries grow, then emerge along Woodlands Trace at 0.5 mile. Keep north beside Woodlands Trace, passing beneath US 68/KY 80. Beyond the road, veer left into a grassy area, shortly reentering woods. Enter a shady pine grove toward a hollow, descending by switchbacks to the upper reaches of Barnett Creek. Cross the streambed then a feeder branch via wooden bridge and reach a trail junction at mile 1.3. The Jenny Ridge Spur Trail leaves right uphill to the Jenny Ridge Picnic Area and Woodlands Trace.

The North–South Trail curves around a bluff, keeping along the Barnett Creek Valley. The streambed's white rocks contrast with the deep green woods. Soon, span another side stream via wooden bridge. The hollow widens, and a small field opens to your right. At mile 2.3, span a bridge over Barnett Creek where two streambeds converge. Here, the Brush Arbor Camp Spur Trail leaves left 0.8 mile to reach a trail shelter, spring, and perennial stream. The North–South Trail curves downstream and follows winding Barnett Creek through bottomland. Bridge a feeder branch, then Barnett Creek itself before reaching Forest Road 143 at mile 2.8.

Cross the forest road and work up a hollow on a singletrack path into hickory-oak woods to split a gap in the ridge. Decline to a feeder branch beside a small field at mile 3.4. Travel a gas pipeline clearing. The pipeline was installed in 1955 and delivers gas from the Gulf of Mexico to states up north.

Pick up a narrow rib ridge to gain your first glimpses of Kentucky Lake through the trees. Reach a gravel promontory at mile 3.9. Here is a small, dry campsite. The North–South Trail descends to come alongside Vickers Bay at mighty Kentucky Lake. This lake, impounded by Kentucky Dam in 1944, is 184 miles long, stretching far south into Tennessee. Keep directly alongside the shoreline. In spring, the North–South Trail may be flooded along the bays. Mountain bikers will have a hard time getting around the flooded bottomlands, but hikers can skirt the waters. Winter will see levels below full pool. Consult the "Fishing" section on pages 32–42 for information about lake levels.

At mile 4.2, span a feeder branch of Vickers Creek. Shortly, come alongside a second bridge and a trail junction. Here, the Dead Beaver Spring Spur Trail leads right 0.8 mile to a reliable spring and campsite. The North–South Trail spans the bridge over Vickers Creek then leads along Vickers Bay. Look for numerous grapevines in the area. LBL's most common vine is the muscadine, enjoyed by wildlife and trail users in late August and September. Pass through a pine plantation and begin the most challenging hills of the trail thus far. Up and down it goes, jumping ridges and dipping into hollows, passing a hillside spring below the trail. Curve away from the lake shortly beyond the spring and join dirt-and-grass FR 338 at mile 5.7. Trace the road for 0.2 mile, then leave left, descending to an unnamed bay at mile 6.3. Views open of Kentucky Lake along the bay. Cross a streambed at the head of the bay. The North–South Trail then passes an old home foundation before bridging the main streambed forming the bay.

Ascend sharply from the unnamed bay on the nose of a ridgeline to join FR 337 at mile 7.2. Keep along the dirt road for 0.3 mile then split left into a pine stand. Leave north along a rolling ridge and drop to Rhodes Bay at mile 8.0. Begin circling the bay to span a creek bed beneath a young forest in the floodplain. Step over the outflow of Buzzard Wing Spring before reaching FR 141 at mile 8.4. Here, the Buzzard Wing Spur Trail leaves right 0.1 mile on FR 141 to a spring and campsite.

The North–South Trail leaves left along FR 141 then dips to a field. Watch carefully at this point, as the North–South Trail splits left from FR 141, crosses Rhodes Creek, and curves left just past a massive multilimbed oak tree. Begin curving around the north side of Rhodes Bay through locust trees reclaiming an old field. The North–South Trail enters a cedar grove until mile 9.0, where it leaves abruptly north, away from Rhodes Bay. Hikers may notice limbs stacked against logs that have fallen across the trail. Mountain bikers do this to make a primitive ramp for jumping over the logs. When the log is removed so are the limbs.

Work over the ridge on double- and singletrack path to reach an arm of Higgins Bay at mile 10.2. Cross a feeder branch, then enjoy views of Higgins Bay from the rocky, hillside path. Dip to a point that overlooks an island just offshore. The old Brown Cemetery stands on this island. The trail hugs the undulating south shore of Higgins Bay. Circle around the floodplain of Higgins Branch, spanning a feeder stream by wooden bridge. Enter a pine thicket, then span Higgins Branch by wooden bridge at mile 11.8. Meander down a wide flat, then climb away from Higgins Bay to reach a trail junction and FR 319 at mile 12.4. Here, the Coffin Cove Spur Trail leads left along rough FR 319, then off the road a bit to Coffin Cove backcountry campsite. Be aware that this campsite has only Kentucky Lake for drinking water. The site does overlook Higgins Bay and has lakeside rocks, providing a convenient entry and exit for swimmers.

The North–South Trail turns right on FR 319, follows it for a quarter mile, then leaves the forest road left on a singletrack path into a hollow. Begin descending along the heavily wooded hollow. Bridge a feeder streambed then the main streambed of the hollow just before reaching FR 140 at mile 13.4. FR 140 leads left a short distance to Sugar Bay Lake Access. The access offers picnic sites and campsites with vault toilets but no potable water.

The North–South Trail crosses FR 140, then ascends a hill. Work around the lake access, reaching a high point, then descend to reach South Fork Sugar Creek at mile 13.9. Several small streams cross the trail in the floodplain. These bridgeless streams flow during more of the year than most LBL streams. Turn away from the flat and pick up an old roadbed beneath a broken canopy. Reach the shoreline of Sugar Bay at mile 14.9. Curve toward the head of the bay to span North Fork Sugar Creek on a long bridge at mile 15.8.

The North–South Trail ascends away from the bay and shortly reaches FR 319. The Pinnegar Cemetery is visible to the left. Turn right on FR 319 and keep climbing to reach a trail junction at mile 16.2. The Sugar Jack Spring Spur Trail leaves right on FR 139, then dips to reach a trail shelter and spring in 1.0 mile. The North–South Trail leaves left on FR 139, following it a quarter mile to a hilltop, then splits right onto a singletrack that follows an old roadbed. Descend toward Duncan Creek Valley. Fields are visible through the trees. Step over a small feeder branch, then a larger stream in bottomland near the fields. The North–South Trail then curves upstream in the valley, keeping fields to your left. Tall tulip trees grow in the margin of woods through which the North–South Trail passes. Reach a trail junction at mile 17.5. Here, the Nature Station Connector Trail leads 4.8 miles to the Nature Station. Notice two very large tulip trees growing directly beside the junction.

The North–South Trail leaves the woods to bisect the agricultural field, crossing Duncan Creek in the middle of the field, then a feeder branch on a high wooden bridge. This stream drains Duncan Lake, a half mile distant. Duncan Lake is popular for eagle viewing in winter. A wooded flat and potential campsite are just beyond the bridge. The North–South Trail then ascends away from the field, traversing a small hill with a wooden bridge over a wet-weather stream before dipping to another dry branch and reaching the Hatchery Hollow backcountry campsite at mile 17.9. Water is available from a hydrant at the nearby wildlife restoration center just uptrail and to the left down a gravel road. The North–South Trail leaves Hatchery Hollow and climbs to reach FR 309 at mile 18.0. This is the end of this trail segment. From here, it is 13.2 miles to the North Welcome Station.

ACCESS   *Golden Pond Trailhead:* Golden Pond Visitor Center is centrally located at LBL. It can be reached from the east on I-24 at Exit 65 via US 68/KY 80, from the north on I-24 from Exit 31 via KY 453 South, from the west by KY 80, and from the south by US 79 and Woodlands Trace. The Golden Pond trailhead is located on Golden Pond Road, the short road that connects Woodlands Trace to US 68/KY 80, just south of the Golden Pond Visitor Center. Look for the gravel parking area beside a few sheltered snack and drink machines.

Duncan Bay Trailhead: From the Golden Pond Visitor Center, take Woodlands Trace north 9.3 miles to FR 132. Turn left on FR 132 and follow it 1.5 miles. Look left for a gated gravel road leading to the old wildlife center. Park on the shoulder of the road leading to the wildlife center. Do not block the gate. The North–South Trail crosses the gravel road just beyond the gate.

■ NORTH–SOUTH TRAIL:
Duncan Bay to North Welcome

LENGTH 13.2 miles   **CONDITION** Mostly good
HIGHS Bluff views of Kentucky Lake, camping opportunities
LOWS Travels along power line for a period   **DIFFICULTY** Moderate
TIPS Hikers and mountain bikers share the trail

THIS FINAL PORTION of trail goes out in grand fashion. It leaves the Duncan Creek Valley, keeping north over a long ridge, then descends to the wide Smith Creek Valley. It works over another ridge to reach the Pisgah Creek Valley, which has campsites ranging from backcountry to more developed sites. Circle around the wide bottomland of Pisgah Creek. Make a long trek along scenic and large Pisgah Bay. The Dodds Creek area offers evidence of old homesites and a trail shelter with a spring. Enter the Hillman Ferry area, which offers a large developed campground before making the final push along the shores of Kentucky Lake, where trail trekkers travel lakeside just above the impoundment and far above on a bluff wooded with oak trees growing over moss and gravel floors.

Begin this trail segment by heading north from the gravel road leading to the closed wildlife restoration center. The white-blazed North–South Trail comes alongside an old fence line—you can see the cedar posts in a line. Descend to cross Forest

Road 309. Just past FR 309 on the right is a nice, flat site suitable for camping. The North–South Trail spans an intermittent creek bed that flows from a spring located upstream about 100 yards. Begin working toward the ridgeline dividing Duncan and Smith creeks. The ascent picks up beyond the Fulks Cemetery on your left. The ridge-top harbors a classic oak forest with moss and gravel groundcover. At mile 1.4, the North–South Trail passes by three wildlife clearings in succession to reach FR 130 at mile 1.9. Turn right on FR 130. A good view opens of the thickly wooded lands to the northeast. Over 90% of LBL's 170,000 acres are forested.

The North–South Trail descends the hill of FR 130 to turn left on the Gray Cemetery access road at mile 2.2. Soon, veer right onto singletrack path, descending to reach the fields of Smith Creek. Stay in the margin of woods and turn north, traversing thickly forested, junglesque bottomland with plentiful river birch trees. Bridge Smith Creek at mile 2.7. Come alongside another field to cross a feeder branch. Here, the North–South Trail leads left into the woods as a singletrack path. Do not keep forward into a clearing.

Curve away from the valley on an incline. At mile 3.5, come alongside a hilltop clearing, then join rough FR 306 leading left through a second meadow. At mile 4.0, leave the forest road heading right, back on singletrack into bottomland laced with small streambeds. The North–South Trail picks up a faint roadbed to reach Old Ferry Road at mile 4.5.

Cross the paved road and head away as a singletrack path, but shortly join a jeep track to dip alongside a massive field. Keep in the margin of woods and walk abreast of the field. Pick up an elevated roadbed to parallel then span Pisgah Creek at mile 5.0. If the water is flowing, this valley makes a good place to camp. Mountain bikers need to watch for the sharp curve before bridging Pisgah Creek.

Cruise in flatwoods to reach a feeder branch of Pisgah Creek and bridge it farther downstream. Reach the shoreline of Pisgah Bay at mile 6.1. Begin a long lakeshore walk. During a wet spring, this part of the trail may be flooded. Birmingham Ferry Campground is visible across the bay. Bridge an unnamed streambed at mile 6.4. A lakeside campsite lies in a mix of grasses and trees near here. Other campsites can be found along the shoreline, but the lake will have to provide your drinking water. The woods become piney just before skirting Pisgah Bay Lake Access. It has picnic sites, campsites, vault toilets, and no water. Climb away from the access to reach Lee Cemetery Road at mile 7.2. Lee Cemetery is visible to your left. Descend from the road around an old homesite on your right. Once heavily settled, look for old fence lines, big trees with widespread limbs, and squared-off flat spots. Over 1,300 homes, containing 5,000 residents, stood during the 1963 announcement of LBL's creation. Most of these homes were demolished, then buried in large excavated holes. Other homes were lifted from their foundations and floated by barge to new sites along the lakes. Those families' sacrifices for the greater recreational good makes LBL appreciated even more.

Dip to a flat and trail junction at mile 7.5. Here, the Nightriders Spring Spur Trail leaves right 0.6 mile to a shelter and spring. The North–South Trail enters a pine grove to span Dodds Creek on a wooden bridge. Keep in mixed pine woods, roaming through dry hills, and come alongside a power line at mile 8.0. Cross the first of three bridges that span creek beds between the hills. The power line clearing stays to your right. Reach paved FR 110 at mile 9.4. It is a half mile left to Hillman Ferry Campground. The campground has hot showers, a telephone, and a small camp store.

Cross FR 110 and begin to ascend through a hickory-oak forest. American elm is an interesting component of this forest. Primarily an understory tree here, American elm ranges from Canada to Texas to Florida to Maine. Look for the elliptical leaves with doubly saw-toothed edges. The bark of this tree is light gray and becomes furrowed in older species. Dutch elm disease, accidentally introduced to the United States in 1930, continues to harm this tree's growth and expansion.

Descend off the hillside to reach the Brown Spring Spur Trail at 10.0 miles. This spur trail leaves right 0.2 mile to a reliable water source. Campsites are in this flat. The North–South Trail soon spans a bridge over the outflow of Brown Spring. Head down the hollow of this streambed, keeping a hill to your right, to reach the embayment of this streambed. Part of Hillman Ferry Campground is visible across the small bay.

The North–South Trail curves around to the main body of Kentucky Lake in a forest of cedar. Pick up an old roadbed and shortly reach the Moss Creek Day-Use Area and FR 109 at mile 10.8. To your left is an attractive gravel beach where folks swim, relax, and fish. The North–South Trail picks up and follows FR 109 over a hill and dips to a low point. Keep your eyes peeled here, as numerous rough jeep roads turn away from FR 109. At mile 11.1, at the low point in the road, the North–South Trail leaves left as a singletrack path. Ascend along this singletrack path and reach a homesite on a hill to your right. Look for the concrete block foundation of the residence.

Climb from the hollow and pick up a bluffline overlooking Kentucky Lake. Attractive oaks growing amid moss grace the edge of the bluff. Begin to curve away from the bluffline toward the embayment of Twin Lakes Lake Access. Circle around the streamshed forming the embayment and reach the lake access. Cross FR 105, which leads to a boat ramp at mile 11.8. Watch for the white blazes leaving right, uphill, and away from the lake access as a singletrack path. Climb to a point overlooking Kentucky Lake then curve past a homesite. Privet, a ground cover planted by the former residents, covers the foundation.

Keep to the right of hollows dipping to the lake and reach gravel FR 104 at mile 12.5. Pass a homesite on your right where the chimney still stands. Cross FR 104 a second time near the northern portion of the Twin Lakes Lake Access. Descend to a streambed and trail junction at 13.0 miles. Here, the Canal Loop Trail has just bridged the streambed and joins the North–South Trail as it keeps north around a potentially wet flat. Meet a paved road then keep right, curving around the North Welcome Station picnic area. Finally, veer left, joining the paved North Paved Trail for the final walk to reach the North Welcome Station and the end of the North–South Trail at mile 13.2.

ACCESS *Duncan Bay Trailhead:* From the Golden Pond Visitor Center, take Woodlands Trace north for 9.3 miles to FR 132. Turn left on FR 132 and follow it for 1.5 miles. Look left for the gated gravel road leading to the old wildlife center. Park on the shoulder of the road leading to the wildlife center. *Do not* block the gate. The North–South Trail crosses the gravel road just beyond the gate.

North Welcome Trailhead: From Exit 31 on I-24 near Lake City, head south on KY 453 7 miles. KY 453 becomes Woodlands Trace once it enters Land Between The Lakes National Recreation Area. The North Welcome Station will be on your right. It can also be reached by heading 20 miles north on Woodlands Trace from the Golden Pond Visitor Center.

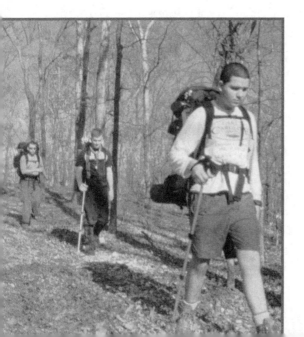

Backpackers on North–South Trail

NORTH–SOUTH TRAIL LOG

0.0   North–South Trail leaves parking area near South Welcome Station

1.0   Turn left at roadbed, soon passing field and pond

2.0   Intersect Fort Henry North–South Connector Trail

2.8   Leave doubletrack wildlife clearing access road

3.9   Stay right near clearing

4.7   Incline leads up to meadow

5.1   Pine plantation

5.3   Stay left at road split

6.0   Trail leads left into pine

6.3   Join rutted gravel track

6.9   Reach Morgan Cemetery and FR 222

7.5   Leave FR 222 on singletrack path

7.9   Brier Rose Branch Spur Trail leads 0.2 mile to spring and campsite

8.1   Cross FR 221

9.0   Fuqua Cemetery on left

9.4   Concrete survey marker to right of trail

10.9   Iron Mountain trail shelter and lookout tower, water near tower
Reach gravel FR 205, Ginger Creek Road

13.9   Model Loop Trail leaves right 0.8 mile to Bison Hideaway campsite

15.2   Spur trail leads 75 yards to Prospectors Place campsite and spring

16.2   Pass clearing with pond

16.8   Intersect north end of Model Loop Trail, cross Woodlands Trace;
begin joint use with equestrians

17.4   Briefly join FR 356

17.7   Enter Kentucky

18.2   Rushing Family Cemetery, then cross Laura Furnace Creek

18.7   Cross FR 165

19.8   Walker Line Trail leads left 2.8 miles to Rushing Creek Campground

20.9   Cross FR 406

22.5   Mountain Laurel Spring Spur Trail leads left 0.8 mile to campsite and spring

23.1 West Fork Laura Furnace Creek; Laura Furnace Fork Spur Trail leads right 0.8 mile to trail shelter and spring

24.1 Cross Fords Bay Road, FR 170

24.6 Reach Colson Overlook Spur Trail after crossing Turkey Creek near spring

25.2 Turkey Spring/School House Hollow Spring Spur Trail leads left to campsite and springs

26.4 Pass behind Compton Cemetery, then join FR 342

27.2 Leave forward away from FR 342, end of joint use with equestrians

28.2 Trace near potable water pump at RV dump station
Golden Pond Spur Trail leads right 0.2 mile to Golden Pond Trailhead

29.1 Come alongside Woodlands Trace, pass under US 68/KY 80

29.9 Jenny Ridge Spur Trail leads right to picnic area and Woodlands Trace

30.9 Bridge Barnett Creek, Brush Arbor Camp Spur Trail leads left 0.8 mile to trail shelter, spring, and perennial stream

31.4 Cross FR 143

32.0 Feeder branch beside small field

32.5 Gravel promontory overlooking Vickers Bay, small, dry campsite

32.8 Span feeder branch on footbridge, reach Dead Beaver Spring Spur Trail that leads right 0.8 mile to reliable spring and campsite, North–South Trail bridges Vickers Creek

34.3 Join FR 338 for 0.2 mile

34.9 Come alongside unnamed bay, views of Kentucky Lake

35.8 Join FR 337 for 0.3 mile

36.6 Reach Rhodes Bay

37.0 Join FR 141; Buzzard Wing Spur Trail leads right to campsite and spring

37.6 Trail abruptly leaves right, away from Rhodes Bay

38.8 Reach arm of Higgins Bay

40.4 Span Higgins Creek on wooden bridge

41.0 Reach FR 319, Coffin Cove Spur Trail leads left 0.2 mile to lakeside campsite

42.0 Cross FR 140, Sugar Bay Lake Access to left

42.5 Cross South Fork Sugar Creek

43.5 Come alongside Sugar Bay

44.4 Long bridge over North Fork Sugar Creek

44.8 Sugar Jack Spring Spur Trail leads right a mile to trail shelter and spring

46.1 Trail junction in Duncan Creek Valley; Nature Station Connector Trail leads right 4.8 miles to Nature Station, North–South Trail crosses agricultural field to reach bridge over Duncan Creek and flat suitable for camping

46.5 Hatchery Hollow campsite, water available from hydrant 0.1 mile distant

46.6 FR 309, end of trail section

47.0 Reach camping flat and spring upstream of wooden bridge after crossing FR 309

48.0 Pass three wildlife clearings in succession

48.5 Reach FR 130, views from hilltop

48.8 Turn left on Gray Cemetery access road; descend to fields of Smith Creek

49.3 Bridge Smith Creek and ascend

50.1 Hilltop clearing, join rough FR 306

50.6 Leave FR 306

51.1 Cross paved Old Ferry Road

51.6 Span Pisgah Creek on bridge

52.7 Reach Shoreline of Pisgah Bay

53.0 Bridge unnamed streambed, lakeside camp nearby

53.8 Cross Lee Cemetery Road after skirting Pisgah Bay Lake Access

54.1 Nightriders Spring Spur Trail leads right to trail shelter and spring

54.6 Come alongside power line

56.0 Cross paved FR 110, Hillman Ferry Campground to left

56.6 Reach Brown Spring Spur Trail in flat; it leads right 0.2 mile to spring

57.4 Pass through Moss Creek Day-Use Area on Kentucky Lake; pick up FR 109

57.7 Trail turns left away from FR 109 on singletrack path

58.4 Cross FR 105

59.1 Cross FR 104

59.6 Intersect Canal Loop Trail

59.8 North Welcome Station, end of trail

North–South Spur Trails

THE NORTH–SOUTH TRAIL is the master path of the Land Between The Lakes trails. The following trails connect the North–South Trail to campsites, springs, trail shelters, trailheads, picnic areas, and campgrounds. While traveling the North–South

Trail, you can consult the following information to learn about the spur trails. "Where" tells what mile of the North–South Trail the spur trail intersects, traveling from south to north. "Length" is the distance of the spur trail, and "Links" tells what the spur trail connects to the North–South Trail.

■ BRIER ROSE SPRING SPUR TRAIL

WHERE Mile 7.9   **LENGTH** 0.2 mile   **LINKS** Brier Rose Spring and campsite

THIS SPUR TRAIL leaves the North–South Trail and descends to a spring in the upper Barrett Creek watershed. Work down along a hill then come to a streambed. Trace the yellow blazes downhill along a streambed to reach the flat. The spring is located in the streambed and will flow in pools for a short distance.

The town of Tharpe was located near here. Back in settler days, Tharpe and other area residents milled flour using water power. However, local streams dried up during the year, rendering water-powered mills inoperable. As modern times came, millers used steam and gas engines to power their mills. A steam-powered mill was opened at Tharpe in 1915. The brand of flour was named Brier Rose and was sold in local stores. It was also shipped in barrels and sacks via the Cumberland River. A red rose was stamped on each sack, inspiring the name for this spring.

■ BROWN SPRING SPUR TRAIL

WHERE Mile 56.8   **LENGTH** 0.2 mile   **LINKS** Brown Spring

THIS SPUR TRAIL leaves the North–South Trail in a streamside flat and runs along a hillside to reach Brown Spring, a reliable water source. Camping is available in the flat near the junction with the North–South Trail. FR 107 is within view of the spring.

The North–South Trail reaches the trail junction at 56.8 miles. Northbound hikers turn right (east) and head up a flat. Potential campsites are here, but more solitude can be found across the streambed near the trail junction. Pass a woodland pond and pick up a hillside to your right. Dip a bit to reach the spring. Part of the spring has been concreted in and covered with a metal grate, but most of the flow emanates from a hillside.

■ BRUSH ARBOR CAMP SPUR TRAIL

WHERE Mile 31.1   **LENGTH** 0.8 mile   **LINKS** Brush Arbor trail shelter and spring

THIS SPUR TRAIL departs from the North–South Trail along Barnett Creek. The path climbs a ridgeline, then drops back into a feeder branch of Barnett Creek to reach a flat, where a metal trail shelter and spring lie. This campsite, though fairly close to US 68/KY 80, exudes remoteness.

Northbound North–South Trail travelers will span Barnett Creek on a wooden bridge then reach the junction with Brush Arbor Camp Spur Trail. Turn left on the yellow-blazed path, heading easterly away from bottomland. Aim toward a ridgeline. The trail climbs onto the wooded ridge. You begin to wonder how a spring is going to be in this unlikely location. The ascent moderates atop the ridge, then dives into a hollow, returning to the bottomland. Cross a feeder branch of Barnett Creek and reach the metal trail shelter at 0.8 mile. The trail continues a short distance beyond the shelter to reach Brush Arbor Spring. It emanates from the hillside beside the shelter and campsite.

The name "Brush Arbor" comes from an old-time practice of pre-LBL residents. Local churches would often hold revival meetings in the summer. These revivals were large events where entire communities would turn out. The churches couldn't hold the crowds, so a brush arbor was constructed to shade folks from the hot sun. Poles were set in the ground and a trellis was constructed. Brush was integrated onto the trellis, allowing breezes in but the sun out. Split logs were placed under the arbor instead of pews. Folks would come and go, listening to the preachers who could sermonize for hours on end. Revival attendees would socialize as well, especially younger people who used these gatherings for courting.

■ BUZZARD WING SPRING SPUR TRAIL

WHERE Mile 37.0   **LENGTH** 0.1 mile   **LINKS** Buzzard Wind Spring and campsite

THIS SPUR TRAIL follows a forest road a short distance then turns up a creek bed to reach a campsite and spring. Both are a little close to the road, but the campsite is attractive. The spring is boxed in and covered with wire. You may need to clear off leaves to access the outflow.

The North–South Trail reaches Forest Road 141 at 37.0 miles. Head right (east) for northbound hikers, and trace the forest road. After a few dips and hills, the yellow-blazed spur trail leaves left from the road toward a creek bed. Pass through a small campsite beneath cedars. The trail continues up the small hollow to reach the spring, backed against a hill beneath a fallen tree.

The term "Buzzard Wing" came from a new type of axe invented by a local resident named Bob Taylor. Timber extraction was on the rise during the early 1900s. Much of the timber was used to make railroad ties that were shipped from the region on the Tennessee River. These ties were hewn by hand. Bob saw a better way to make an axe for hewing ties. He called it a "Buzzard Wing" axe, which was patented and officially named the "Keen Kutter."

■ COFFIN COVE SPUR TRAIL

WHERE Mile 41.0   **LENGTH** 0.2 mile   **LINKS** Coffin Cove campsite on Higgins Bay

NORTH-SOUTH TRAIL TREKKERS who want to camp on the shores of Kentucky Lake will use this trail to access a backcountry campsite on Higgins Bay of Kentucky Lake. The name Coffin Cove was inspired by the making of coffins by former LBL homesteaders. When a neighbor passed away, nearby residents used the ample timber supply of the area to build a coffin for the recently deceased. Other residents took up coffin making as a side trade. Coffins were also sold in general stores. In one odd instance, a doctor made coffins on the side.

Reach the Coffin Cove Spur Trail at mile 41.0 of the North–South Trail. Northbound trail trekkers will turn left onto rough Forest Road 319 and ascend a low hill on the yellow-blazed trail. Dip from the hill and look left, as the trail leads down to Higgins Bay. A fire ring stands in an open area near the shore. A suitable, level tent site lies beneath trees to your right as you face the bay. A few exposed rocks on the shoreline make entering the water for a swim easier. Take note that campers will have to haul in their water or treat water from the lake for use.

■ COLSON OVERLOOK SPUR TRAIL

WHERE Mile 24.6   **LENGTH** 0.4 mile   **LINKS** Colson Overlook Picnic Area

THIS TRAIL LEAVES the North–South Trail and ascends from the upper Turkey Creek Valley to a knob where the Colson Overlook Picnic Area stands. A far-reaching vista of Kentucky Lake can be gained from this overlook.

Northbound North–South Trail hikers will cross Turkey Creek at mile 24.6, just before reaching a trail junction. The unsigned Colson Overlook Spur Trail makes an acute left turn. This trail turns back up the maple- and tulip-tree-studded valley before shortly reaching a wet weather feeder branch forming a hollow. The trail heads into this hollow, ascending along the branch. Shortly, leave the streambed and pick up a finger ridge, climbing steeply. The trail levels off in oak woods and reaches a small pond and equestrian picnic area. Make a final climb onto a grassy hill beside a pine plantation to reach the main picnic area and Woodlands Trace at 0.4 mile. Across Woodlands Trace, to your west, Kentucky Lake is visible in the distance.

■ DEAD BEAVER SPRING SPUR TRAIL

WHERE Mile 33.0   **LENGTH** 0.8 mile   **LINKS** Dead Beaver Spring and camp

THE NAME DEAD Beaver Spring doesn't sound too appealing, but it has historical significance. First, LBL backpackers weren't the first to camp here. Archaeological crews from Murray State University found an older campsite just east of the spring. Archaic hunters, the ancients, periodically camped here from 4000 to 1000 BC. These hunters came here now and then, using the site as a butchering ground to process their kills. Stone knives, scrapers, and other tools were found at this site that the archaeologists dubbed Dead Beaver Site.

Historical import of this site notwithstanding, it is a bit of a haul, mostly along a forest road, to reach this spring. If Vickers Creek—near the junction of this spur trail—is flowing, I recommend getting water out of it. The spring and campsite are too close to the forest road.

Heading north on the North–South Trail, pick up the yellow-blazed Dead Beaver Spring Spur Trail just before the wooden bridge over Vickers Creek, at mile 33.0. Turn right on the spur trail, heading upstream along Vickers Creek. At 0.1 mile, emerge onto Forest Road 141. The spur trail follows the forest road right, keeping a large field to your right.

Trace the winding forest road, and at 0.8 mile, the trail leaves the road left. Walk 40 yards off the road to reach the spring at the confluence of two small branches. The camp is between the spring and the road.

■ FORT HENRY NORTH–SOUTH TRAIL CONNECTOR

WHERE Mile 2.0   **LENGTH** 1.4 miles   **LINKS** Fort Henry Trail System, also part of Bear Creek Loop

THIS IMPORTANT SPUR trail enables hikers to combine the North–South Trail with the 29 miles of the Fort Henry Trail System and, in combination with the Telegraph and North–South Trails, makes for one of the best loop hikes at LBL.

The Fort Henry North–South Connector Trail is nothing special in and of itself. It simply courses the Tennessee Divide, which separates the Cumberland and Tennessee River watersheds. In this case, Panther Creek and the Tennessee River are to the west. Bear Creek and the Cumberland River are to the east.

At 2.0 miles on the North–South Trail, the yellow-blazed connector trail leaves left. It climbs a small hill then undulates along the ridgeline, occasionally passing pine stands planted for wildlife cover and erosion breaks. Open into a small meadow, then reenter woods. Break into a second, larger meadow. Pass through the center of the meadow and reach paved Fort Henry Road at 0.8 mile. Keep forward on dirt Forest Road 399, passing a small pond on your right. The dirt road soon ends—reenter woods on a wide trail. Undulate to reach a trail junction at mile 1.4. Here, the Telegraph Trail leads left 3.2 miles to the picnic area near the South Welcome Station and right 4.3 miles to the Fort Henry trailhead.

■ FERRY LANDING SPUR TRAIL

WHERE Mile 51.3   **LENGTH** 1.0 mile   **LINKS** Backcountry campsite nearby and water access to Birmingham Ferry Campground

THIS SPUR TRAIL leads away from the North–South Trail to a hilltop campsite near Kentucky Lake. Birmingham Ferry Campground and its year-round water pump are just down the hill. Northbound hikers will leave the North–South Trail at mile 51.3, turning left on paved Forest Road 114, Old Ferry Road. Follow the road southwest. Yellow blazes are infrequent. At 0.5 mile, veer right off the paved road and trace the yellow blazes onto a settler road in woodland. Top out on a hill and stay left, as a faint roadbed leaves right. At 0.9 mile, atop a hill, reach a level area that serves as a no-cost campsite. The Ferry Landing Trail continues past the camp and descends to a road at Birmingham Ferry Campground. Turn right down the road to reach a water spigot. Fee camping is available at Birmingham Ferry.

It was at Birmingham Ferry that the last Shawnee Indians of the area were loaded onto boats and sent west via the Tennessee River after the Indian Removal Act of 1830. Back in the old days, bridges did not connect the peninsula between the Cumberland and Tennessee Rivers that is now LBL. Ferries were used to cross the rivers and were located at various points along the rivers. Fees were charged according to what was crossing the river, be it a man on a horse or a family in a wagon. Some ferries continued operating even after bridges linked the area in the 1930s. The last ferry in the area shut down in 1964. A ferry operates to this day in Cumberland City, Tennessee, about 20 miles southeast of LBL. The ferry crosses the Cumberland River.

■ GOLDEN POND SPUR TRAIL

WHERE Mile 28.6   **LENGTH** 0.2 mile   **LINKS** Golden Pond trailhead and visitor center

THIS TRAIL LINKS the North–South Trail with the Golden Pond Visitor Center and trailhead. The yellow-blazed Golden Pond Spur Trail leaves east from the North–South Trail to immediately cross Woodlands Trace. It then enters a patch of woods and splits at 0.1 mile. Here, one trail leaves right to shortly reach the Golden Pond trailhead, which has snack and drink machines, a portable toilet, and a telephone. The other trail tops a hill. It then turns right to reach the Golden Pond Visitor Center, which offers informative and historical displays, and has telephones, water, and drink machines. On the far side of the visitor center is Golden Pond. Many theories abound as to how it got its name, from the color of the water, to gold fish in the water, to gold planted around the pond by an unscrupulous realtor.

■ JENNY RIDGE SPUR TRAIL

WHERE Mile 30.1   **LENGTH** 0.2 mile   **LINKS** Jenny Ridge Picnic Area

THIS SHORT TRAIL climbs a hill to reach a picnic area atop Jenny Ridge. After leaving the Golden Pond area, northbound North–South hikers will reach an unsigned trail junction at the head of Barnett Creek. The yellow-blazed Jenny Ridge Spur Trail leaves east from the North–South Trail. It curves uphill from the upper Barnett Creek Valley into a dry oak forest on a rocky path, reaching the Jenny Ridge Picnic Area at 0.2 mile. Picnic tables, grills, and a portable toilet are located here beside Woodlands Trace.

■ LAURA FURNACE FORK SPUR TRAIL

WHERE Mile 23.1, 24.1   **LENGTH** 1.6 miles   **LINKS** Laura Furnace Fork spring and trail shelter

THIS TRAIL LEAVES the North–South Trail and heads along West Fork Laura Furnace Creek before crossing the creek and following a feeder stream beside a pine plantation and fields to reach Laura Furnace Fork spring and trail shelter. This metal shelter stands in a flat beside a pair of springs providing water for backpackers. The yellow-blazed path then climbs steeply away from the springs to an oak-covered ridge. It then passes a hilltop field before reaching Forest Road 170, Fords Bay Road, which the path briefly follows before reuniting with the North–South Trail. This can be combined with the North–South Trail for a good loop hike starting from Fords Bay Road.

Northbound hikers meet this spur trail at mile 23.1 of the North–South Trail. Northbound hikers will make an acute right turn, heading downstream along West Fork Laura Furnace Creek. The creek's namesake, Laura Furnace, was the last iron ore furnace to be built in what was known then as Between The Rivers. The year was 1855. Over 130 workers were used in the 6,000-acre furnace land holding: timber cutters, charcoal makers, limestone extractors, furnace operators, and others. The outbreak of the Civil War stopped the profitable operation. Postwar profits were insufficient for continued operations, and the Laura Furnace cast its last iron in 1872, leaving only a name for a creek.

Keep along the twisting West Fork Laura Furnace Creek as the yellow-blazed trail widens when it picks up a field access road. Reach a junction at 0.3 mile. Turn left here and cross the creek, now with Wranglers Trail 6, which designates a horse trail emerging from Wranglers Campground. Follow the wide path beside a small field to your right. Ahead, the path comes alongside a pine plantation on your right. Shortly, step over a streambed and parallel a narrow field. These bottomland fields are typically

Author at the Laura Furnace shelter on the North–South Trail

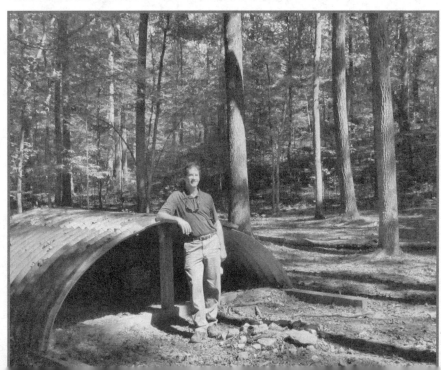

planted with sunflowers or corn. Private farmers work these fields and leave a certain amount of the crop for wildlife in exchange for using the land.

Reach a confusing area at 0.6 mile. Wranglers Trail 6 curves right around a pine stand. The Laura Furnace Fork Spur Trail stays left to cross an intermittent streambed and opens to a second narrow field. Look for the yellow blazes as the path shifts into the woods to the right of the field. Keep parallel to the narrow field on the foot trail, ignoring any trails that turn away from the field. The trail curves left around the west end of the field, reaching Laura Furnace Fork Spring at 0.8 mile. Here is a level spot for camping and a metal trail shelter. The shelter overlooks the last field. The spring run flows beside the shelter. The second spring is just across the spring run.

Laura Furnace Fork Spur Trail crosses the spring run and climbs steeply onto a rib ridge dominated by chestnut oak. The climb eases once atop the ridge. Approach a field on your right but stay in the woods. Reach Fords Bay Road at mile 1.5. Turn left on the gravel road and soon reach the North–South Trail.

■ MODEL LOOP TRAIL

WHERE Mile 13.7, 16.8   **LENGTH** 7.4-mile loop total, including North–South portion of loop
LINKS Bison Hideaway campsite and spring, Bison Range, Homeplace trailhead

THIS TRAIL DESCRIPTION starts at The Homeplace trailhead rather than one of its two junctions with the North–South Trail. Most folks hiking this loop begin here when doing the whole loop. To access The Homeplace trailhead from the South Welcome Station, take Woodlands Trace 10.6 miles north to The Homeplace. Just after turning right into The Homeplace, turn left on the gravel road before crossing the bridge into the paved parking area. Follow the gravel road left 60 yards to reach The Homeplace trailhead. The Model Loop Trail leaves north from the trailhead, following the yellow blazes.

Start at The Homeplace trailhead and cross Woodlands Trace to reach the northeastern end of the Bison Range, a meadow where buffalo live where they did hundreds of years ago between the Tennessee and Cumberland Rivers. Then head north to reach the North–South Trail. Meander along the high, oak-covered ridge dividing these two river watersheds, visiting wildlife clearings, a spring, and a homesite along the way before parting ways with the North–South Trail. Return to the Bison Range and skirt its border for over 2 miles, where you are sure to see some of the large shaggy creatures. Much of the trail is exposed, especially along the Bison Range.

The name "Model" in Model Loop is after the town that was once here. First named Bass after the first postmaster here in 1846, Bass became Great Western when the iron furnace fired up in 1854 just south of here. The post office ceased operations shortly after the furnace closed in 1856 due to a slave insurrection. The whole area was chaos during the Civil War, but the community was still determined to be a success, deciding to later name themselves Model—as in the model town that it wanted to be. The government bought out Model, like many other communities, when LBL was established in the 1960s.

Leave The Homeplace trailhead, walking north on a path blazed in yellow rectangles. Immediately cross Prior Creek, which usually runs dry at this crossing. If you cannot make it across Prior Creek, abandon the hike, because if Prior Creek is running high, so are other streams you will have difficulty crossing. The Model Loop Trail enters a brushy area returning to forest, then reaches broken pine-cedar woods. The grass is mown a little lower along the trailway. Broken pavement indicates this area was settled. Near a well, surrounded by a metal fence, climb a small, grassy hill. Descend to Woodlands Trace, but don't cross it yet—keep north along the paved road beside shortleaf pines. Cross Woodlands Trace, then come to the northeastern end of the Bison Range near a large auto sign indicating the Bison Range. Keep forward just a bit, then span a wooden bridge over a feeder branch of Prior Creek at 0.4 mile.

Keep with the yellow blazes, ascending along the feeder branch, which breaks up in often-dry rivulets. Continue north, straddling the margin between the dry, oak-clad hill to your left and the moisture-loving trees, such as maple, to your right. Cross the main streambed at 0.8 mile. Moss and ferns line the narrow and deep ravine-like streambed. The hollow narrows and hills close in. Rise to meet the North–South Trail at mile 1.5. To your right is a dirt road reaching Woodlands Trace. Ahead is the northbound portion of the North–South Trail. Turn left on the southbound part of the North–South Trail. This is the Tennessee Divide, the high line separating the Tennessee and Cumberland Rivers. Streams to your left flow to the Cumberland River. Streams to your right flow to the Tennessee River.

White rectangular blazes generally mark the North–South Trail. Immediately pass the remains of an old jalopy on your right. The North–South Trail soon enters a linear, grassy wildlife clearing straddling the top of the ridgeline. Briefly reenter woods before reaching a second wildlife clearing at mile 2.1. These wildlife clearings enhance feeding opportunities by creating different growth environments for more natural edibles. A wildlife pond lies to the left of the trail.

Reenter woods and ascend away from the field on a slightly gullied track. At mile 2.7, pass along the left-hand side of another wildlife clearing. Old roads spur from the main trail bed—watch for the white blazes. Wind along the ridgeline, shooting for small gaps and curving along hills. Descend to cross a streambed. At 3.2 miles, reach a yellow-blazed side trail leading right. This trail leads a short distance to the Prospectors Place homesite and spring. A crumbled stone chimney, washtubs, and other relics mark the backcountry campsite.

The North–South Trail ascends away from the side trail up a gullied old roadbed to reach a wildlife clearing with watering hole at mile 4.1. Pass through the clearing into woods and meet a trail junction at mile 4.5. The North–South Trail continues forward. The Model Loop Trail, however, veers acutely left, easterly, toward Bison Hideaway backcountry campsite. Bisect a fast-disappearing clearing and, at mile 4.7, watch for the trail to drop right, off the jeep track it has been tracing. It briefly dips into a hollow, then picks up a less obvious roadbed. Descend off the ridgeline to reach the Bison Range fence at mile 5.3. To your right is a park maintenance area. The Model Loop Trail turns left. Just ahead, a yellow-blazed spur trail leads left to the Bison Hideaway backcountry campsite. The campsite is located 75 yards into the trees beside a streambed.

The Model Loop Trail keeps along the fence line, crossing the streambed via culvert. The path no longer follows yellow blazes but stays with the mown fence perimeter. Climb up over a couple of steep hills offering a view of the Bison Range and the Great Western Iron Furnace to the southeast. To your left, the woods have been cleared away then burned in an effort to enhance wildlife viewing and keep trees from falling onto the fence, which would allow the buffalo to escape. Buffalo will be spotted eventually, depending upon which area they are located.

Buffalo once roamed in vast herds among the prairie grasses of Kentucky and Tennessee. The American bison was a valuable source of food and comfort to the first Americans and to the settlers who came after. Buffalo were a store on hooves to these early LBL residents, providing warm robes and blankets. They also aided in transportation, as the large herds made wide trails along the easiest paths between destinations and to water. Unregulated hunting was a way of life for early settlers in America. Later, as animals became valued more for their hides than their meat, several species in the area became threatened, including elk, bison, and white-tailed deer. By 1846, unregulated hunting and loss of habitat caused the loss of elk and bison in Kentucky and Tennessee.

As early as 1969, TVA initiated efforts to restore bison in LBL. Today, because of the cooperation of several state, local, and federal organizations, and private individuals, there are two bison herds at LBL. The herd you will see here is known as the south herd. The other herd can be seen along with the restored elk in the Elk & Bison Prairie near Golden Pond Visitor Center.

At LBL, an adult buffalo requires about four acres of land to provide adequate forage. The herd is reduced annually to prevent overgrazing in the pasture. As the herd reaches carrying capacity, buffalo are sold to keep the herd in balance with the range. Be careful around these big critters—they are quick and agile. Buffalo appear relatively docile, but they can be unpredictable and dangerous. Do not approach or provoke them.

Keep north beyond your viewing hill as the Model Trail crosses a rocky branch then levels off. Pass a corral on your right at mile 6.1. Hikers can cut between the fences to reach Woodlands Trace. These fences divide the range in two. Cross a large, intermittent feeder stream of Prior Creek just ahead. The trail turns sharply left here. Note the huge, streamside sycamore tree. Keep forward, walking the open margin between the range fence and the wooded creek bed. At mile 6.5, begin curving around the far, west end of the range. Climb one last hill that offers more panoramic views of the field and the watering pond below. Descend to reach a trail junction at mile 7.0. You will recognize this junction at the northeastern end of the Bison Range. Cross Woodlands Trace and backtrack 0.4 mile to reach The Homeplace trailhead.

■ MOUNTAIN LAUREL SPRING SPUR TRAIL

WHERE Mile 22.5   **LENGTH** 0.8 mile
LINKS Mountain Laurel Spring and backcountry campsite

THIS PATH LEAVES the North–South Trail and crosses over to the west side of Woodlands Trace into upper Redd Hollow to reach a quality spring and backcountry campsite. Along the way, it passes through one of the largest stands of mountain laurel in LBL. Mountain laurel is primarily found in the Tennessee River drainage of the recreation area if it is found at all.

Leave the North–South Trail on the spur trail and walk northwest through oak woods, soon coming to a gullied intermittent branch. The fern-lined gully is 8–10 feet deep in places. Shortly, pass beside a pine plantation, then through a wet area wooded with maples. The Mountain Laurel Spring Spur Trail reaches Woodlands Trace. Veer right, crossing Woodlands Trace just beyond Forest Road 167. Reenter woods, keeping north alongside Woodlands Trace. Look left for a small bluff that overlooks a pit. Gravel was once mined here, likely for area roads.

At 0.5 mile, Woodlands Trace and the spur trail turn away from each other. Drop down the rocky path flanked with mountain laurel. The shrubby evergreen is more common in the eastern mountains of Kentucky and Tennessee. In Redd Hollow, reach a trail junction shaded by sweet gum, sycamore, and maple. To your right, a yellow-blazed spur trail leads about 50 yards to the Mountain Laurel Spring back-country campsite. The campsite is set in a small flat beside an intermittent stream. FR 167 is visible through the trees. The spring trail crosses the main branch of Redd Hollow, then reaches FR 167.

Walk down FR 167 a short distance and look left for the trail as it heads up the narrow hollow created by the spring. The path soon ends at the outflow, which emerges below a tree. Mountain Laurel Spring was once boxed in and had a wire cover, but this setup has deteriorated. The water, however, is cool, clear, and inviting.

■ NIGHTRIDERS SPRING SPUR TRAIL

WHERE Mile 54.1   **LENGTH** 0.6 mile   **LINKS** Nightriders Spring and trail shelter

THIS SIDE TRAIL works up a flat along Dodds Creek, then crosses Dodds Creek via a forest service road. It then picks up an old farm road to reach a metal shelter and spring.

Northbound North–South Trail travelers will reach the trail junction with the Nightriders Spring Spur Trail at mile 54.1. Turn right on the yellow-blazed spur trail, walking away from a pine grove. Travel easterly in the margin between a hillside to your right and a thicket of spindly hardwoods to your left. Overhead are wild cherry, tulip, and maple trees in addition to ever-present oaks, some large. Leave this pretty area and reach Forest Road 111 at 0.3 mile. Turn left on FR 111, passing under a power line and over Dodds Creek on the road bridge. Look for a large oak beside the forest road and turn right onto an old farm road. Pass around the cable gate. Note the rusty wire fence along the edge of the farm road. Reach the metal trail shelter in a flat backed against a steep hill. Dodds Creek is nearby. The trail continues along the farm road just a short distance to reach Nightriders Spring on the edge of Dodds Creek.

The Night Riders were a group of tobacco farmers who attempted to scare other tobacco farmers into joining the Tobacco Planters Protective Association of Kentucky and Tennessee. In the early 1900s, a company known as the Tobacco Trust was dominating the tobacco market, especially with what was known as dark tobacco. The Tobacco Trust offered to purchase tobacco at what the farmers deemed a cheap price. So the farmers formed the association to force Tobacco Trust to buy at association prices. Not all area farmers joined the association. The Night Riders threatened the holdouts, eventually resorting to destroying private property, includ-ing barns, tobacco fields, and farm equipment, in what became known as the Dark Tobacco War. In 1907, this culminated in the burning of Golden Pond's only tobacco warehouse. The warehouse owner, an independent dealer from Tennessee, lost 8,000 pounds of tobacco.

■ SUGAR JACK SPRING SPUR TRAIL

WHERE Mile 44.8   **LENGTH** 1.0 mile   **LINKS** Sugar Jack Spring and trail shelter

THIS SPUR TRAIL leaves the North–South Trail high on a ridge and mostly follows forest roads to reach a feeder branch of North Fork Sugar Creek and a trail shelter. The name "Sugar Jack" is an old-time nickname for whiskey.

Heading north on the North–South Trail, reach a junction at mile 44.8. Leave right, easterly, on the yellow-blazed Sugar Jack Spring Spur Trail along Forest Road 139. Follow this ridgetop road for 0.5 mile, then turn right onto FR 318, dropping steeply off the ridge. Step over a streambed and climb a smaller hill. Pass a stock pond on the right as you open to a field. The trail descends to a second streambed. Turn left off the forest road just before reaching the streambed. Here, the trail heads upstream along the watercourse through lush woods. The streambed is littered with limestone rocks. The stream curves left ahead. Step over the streambed and come to Sugar Jack Spring, which is boxed in and covered with wire. Ahead and to the left is the trail shelter. The shelter is set on a slight slope beneath a large shagbark hickory and other trees.

Remains of a still were found near this spring, and sugar is a major ingredient in making the mash that is distilled in producing the whiskey, thus the shelter's nickname. Whiskey is clear when it is first distilled. The oak barrels in which it is aged give the brownish-red color. Oak barrels were made primarily of white oak, of which there are plenty in LBL. Whiskey made in the Golden Pond area was very popular during and after the Prohibition era.

■ TURKEY SPRING/SCHOOL HOUSE HOLLOW SPRING SPUR TRAIL

WHERE Mile 25.2   **LENGTH** 0.6 mile   **LINKS** Turkey Spring and campsite, School House Hollow Spring

THIS SPUR TRAIL leaves the North–South Trail in the Turkey Creek bottoms. It then passes by a cemetery and reaches School House Hollow, where a neat and very reliable rocked-in spring emerges from a hillside. The spur trail continues down a forest road then turns into a hollow where attractive Turkey Spring and campsite lie.

Leave the North–South Trail at mile 25.2. The yellow-blazed spur trail ascends a hill to reach Forest Road 413. Turkey Creek Cemetery is within sight to the left. The spur trail keeps forward and dips to reach a hollow at 0.3 mile. To the right of the road is a flat suitable for camping. The trail passes through the camping area then curves right, toward a hillside where School House Hollow Spring emerges from a rocked-in culvert.

More than a century ago, a schoolhouse stood near here. The log building doubled as a church on Sunday. Consider the students and worshipers who drank from this spring before the building burned around 1900. Today, car campers sometimes set up in School House Hollow. Backpackers seeking solitude should continue down FR 413 0.2 mile farther. The yellow-blazed spur trail heads into the next hollow, on the right beyond School House Hollow, as a singletrack path just across a road leading into a field on the left. If you pass water flowing over FR 413, you have gone too far. Trace the singletrack path up the hollow over a small footbridge to shortly reach the spring and campsite. The small campsite feels remote. The screened-in spring emerges from a hillside to the right of the campsite.

■ WALKER LINE TRAIL

WHERE Mile 19.8   **LENGTH** 2.8 miles   **LINKS** Rushing Creek Campground

DEPENDING ON WHICH direction you go, this trail connects Kentucky to Tennessee or vice versa. The state line is important here, as it relates to the name of the trail. More about that later. The North–South Trail is on the northeast terminus of the Walker Line Trail. Backpackers often trek the 60-plus miles of the North–South Trail end to end. Rushing Creek Campground is on the southwest end of the Walker Line Trail. From April through October, Rushing Creek operates hot showers. Dirty North–South Trail backpackers will use the Walker Line Trail to access Rushing Creek, enjoying the attractive lakeside campground and hot showers. Campers at Rushing Creek will hike the Walker Line Trail to the North–South Trail, then come back and take a shower.

This description is from Rushing Creek Campground area to the North–South Trail. To reach this end of the trail from the South Welcome Station, take Woodlands Trace 13 miles north to paved Forest Road 172. Turn left and follow FR 172 for 2.1 miles. Look on your right for the yellow-blazed trail. Continue driving a short piece to the parking area on the left where FR 172 splits, with Rushing Creek Camping Area to the left and Jones Creek Camping Area to the right. Park here and backtrack down FR 172 to begin the trail.

Leave north from FR 172 and begin walking the Walker Line Trail. Cruise through hickory-oak woods, dip in a swale, and reach the state line at 0.5 mile. You have left Stewart County, Tennessee, and are now in Trigg County, Kentucky. The exact line seems trivial now. However, during the Civil War, Tennessee was part of the Confederacy and Kentucky was neutral. Before the war, local citizens weren't sure which state they were in, much less the roaming Union soldiers and Confederate guerrillas who came later, looking for sympathizers loyal to the other side.

Back in the late 1700s, Tennessee was part of North Carolina and Kentucky was part of Virginia. Virginia and North Carolina couldn't agree on the exact boundary between the two states. So Virginia hired Dr. Thomas Walker to survey their southern border, which was supposed to run along 36 degrees, 30 minutes latitude. By the time Walker reached the Tennessee River, he was about 17 miles north of the latitude line. Later, when Kentucky became a state in 1792, it rejected Walker's survey, but Tennessee, which became a state in 1796, stood by the line. As the Civil War became imminent, the disputed line, the Walker Line, effectively became the border between the states.

Work around a former field just past the state line. The canopy stays open as often as not on the ensuing trailway. The yellow blazes trace the old logging road as it passes a nearly dried-out stock pond on the left. Reach Woodlands Trace at mile 1.4. Turn left, heading north along the paved highway. Pass a field on your right at mile 1.8. Continue along Woodlands Trace to mile 2.0. Here, turn right off Woodlands Trace onto the gravel road, leading right toward Bullock Cemetery. Follow the gravel road through oak woods mixed with a sprinkling of pine and cedar to reach the North–South Trail at mile 2.2. From here, the North–South Trail heads north 9.0 miles to Golden Pond and south 20 miles to the South Welcome Station. If you are walking this trail from the North–South Trail to Rushing Creek, be advised that Rushing Creek campground is 0.6 mile west on FR 172 from where the Walker Line Trail emerges onto FR 172, for a total of 2.8 miles from the North–South Trail.

Wranglers Trails

THE WRANGLERS TRAILS are a group of bridle paths that emanate from Wranglers Camp, a campground for equestrians. This trail system uses numbered and named trails, though most riders refer to the trail by its number and not its name. Although the Wranglers Trails are not reserved exclusively for equestrians, it is recommended that only equestrians use them. These paths, generally wider than hiking trails at LBL, have been designed for horse and horse-drawn wagon use. LBL horseback riders have the greater Lick Creek area as their domain over which these nearly

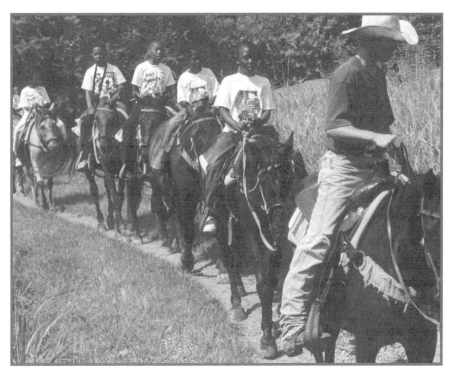

Wranglers; photo courtesy of TVA

100 miles of path cover. The Wranglers Trails sometimes follow gravel roads or go alongside a few paved roads in LBL. The trails also trace the shoreline of Lake Barkley and roam atop hickory-oak ridges, through wide fields, and in valleys. Many equestrians simply piddle around the campground roads.

Bicyclers are expressly forbidden from using the Wranglers Trails to prevent accidents and to avoid frightening the horses. Hikers have other trail choices better suited to enhance their experience. Be aware that a section of the North–South Trail is open to horses and hikers. The condition of each individual trail is dependent on recent precipitation and repair. Winter and spring can be muddy, as can summer after thunderstorms. Late summer and fall see the driest trail conditions.

Black numbers mark the trails. They are generally placed onto trees at eye level of a horseback rider. Other markers are placed on posts. An arrow indicating which direction the trail travels usually accompanies the trail number. Equestrians will undoubtedly notice "bootleg trails," unauthorized paths that shortcut legal trails. Please avoid using these paths, as they are not maintained and cause erosion that harms area watersheds and legal trails. The forest service has a hard enough time keeping the legal trails maintained. Wranglers Trail maps, including trail descriptions, are available at the North Welcome Station, South Welcome Station, Golden Pond Visitor Center, and online, in addition to Wranglers Campground.

ACCESS From the entrance of Golden Pond Visitor Center, take Woodlands Trace south 0.2 mile to paved Forest Road 165. Turn left on FR 165 and follow it 5.0 miles to an intersection. FR 166 keeps forward. Turn right here, as FR 165 shortly reaches Wranglers Campground.

Suggested Loops

HIKING LOOPS

WHAT FOLLOWS ARE suggested loop hikes in each of the major divisions of the recreation area. To find the trailhead, simply look at the first trail listed in the "Trails Used" information. Use the trails in the order they are listed. "Difficulty" is for average hikers, "Length" is the mileage of the trail portions in the loop, and "Highlights" indicates what is of interest along the way.

Tennessee

■ BEAR CREEK LOOP

TRAILS USED Telegraph Trail, Fort Henry North–South Trail Connector, North–South Trail
DIFFICULTY Moderate   LENGTH 6.6 miles
HIGHLIGHTS Spring wildflowers, homesites, varied terrain

THIS LOOP, ONE of the best at LBL, leaves the picnic area across at the intersection of Woodlands Trace and Fort Henry Road just north of the South Welcome Station. Head south on the Telegraph Trail. Dip into the Bear Creek watershed among some of the best wildflower displays at LBL. Pass old homesites and fields along Dry Branch before climbing onto a ridgeline. Turn north on the Fort Henry North–South Trail Connector past meadows to meet the North–South Trail. Return to the picnic area after passing through an attractive woodland.

■ MODEL LOOP TRAIL

TRAILS USED Model Loop Trail, North–South Trail
DIFFICULTY Moderate   LENGTH 7.4 miles
HIGHLIGHTS Bison Range, springs, old homesite

THIS LOOP LEAVES The Homeplace trailhead and crosses Woodlands Trace to reach the Bison Range and then the North–South Trail. At the North–South Trail the loop turns southerly along Tennessee Ridge and cruises past many wildlife clearings, then the old Prospectors Place homesite and spring. Return to the Bison Range and follow its perimeter for over 2.0 miles before completing the loop. A detailed description of this trail is included in the "North–South Spur Trails" section on pages 131–134.

■ PICKET LOOP

TRAILS USED Boswell Trail, Picket Loop Trail   **DIFFICULTY** Moderate
LENGTH 3.6 miles   **HIGHLIGHTS** Kentucky Lake vistas, old homesites

THIS LOOP IS the most northwesterly trail in the Fort Henry Trail System. Leave the Fort Henry trailhead to circle a ridgeline and drop down along Kentucky Lake near Panther Bay, passing a couple of interesting homesites. Walk along the shoreline of Kentucky Lake before climbing into a young oak forest to complete the loop. A detailed description of this trail is included in the "Fort Henry Trails" section on pages 87–89.

■ RIVER CIRCLE/DONELSON LOOP

TRAILS USED Donelson Trail, River Circle Trail
DIFFICULTY Moderate to difficult   **LENGTH** 2.1 miles
HIGHLIGHTS Steep wooded ravines, big trees, view of Lake Barkley from river batteries

THIS GREAT LOOP takes place at Fort Donelson National Battlefield. Start at Jackson's Battery and take the Donelson Trail as it immediately descends into a steep, pretty hollow that is home to some huge trees. Climb out of this hollow only to drop into a second hollow. Keep toward Lake Barkley to meet the River Circle Trail. Make sure to walk out to the river batteries, where cannon emplacements overlook the dammed Cumberland River. Return via the River Circle Trail, which also has many steep ups and downs in scenic hollows.

Kentucky

■ ADMIN LOOP

TRAILS USED Admin Trail, North–South Trail, Golden Pond Spur Trail
DIFFICULTY Easy   **LENGTH** 1.4 miles
HIGHLIGHTS Convenient loop from Golden Pond Visitor Center

THIS LOOP WINDS around the immediate Golden Pond Visitor Center area. Its beginning is the Administration Trail—the "Admin Trail," as LBL employees know it. This trail originated in response to a national energy crisis. Back during the gasoline wars of the 1970s, when the Tennessee Valley Authority (TVA) ran LBL, TVA officials decided to cut fuel usage by employees. They built this trail connecting the visitor center, the administration building, and the maintenance building so that employees could walk or bicycle between buildings. Later, the gasoline crisis passed, but the trail remained. And to this day employees use the trail for work and exercise. Somewhere along the line, the term "Admin Trail" was coined. Now, you can walk this path and make a loop, in conjunction with the North–South Trail, to get a little taste of LBL.

Take the Admin Trail as it leaves the visitor center. Walk out the back door and look for the paved trail leading from the building. Walk a few steps and turn left, following the paved trail. (The paved trail leading forward is your return route.) The Administration Trail dips along a wet-weather stream in a line of trees. At 0.2 mile, the trail tunnels beneath Golden Pond Road. Keep in thick woods. The uppermost valley of Elbow Creek is below to your left. The trail curves around the administration building, passing an employee picnic area. Cross a gravel road to emerge onto paved Forest Road 165. Follow the forest road right to reach Woodlands Trace. Turn left on Woodlands Trace and cross the road. Look right for the North–South Trail as it reenters the woods after crossing Woodlands Trace. The North–South Trail curves back to the north through oak woods to reach the Golden Pond Spur Trail. The yellow-blazed Golden Pond Spur Trail leaves east from the North–South Trail to immediately cross Woodlands Trace. Stay left after crossing Woodlands Trace and return to the rear of the visitor center.

■ HONKER TRAIL

TRAILS USED Honker Trail
DIFFICULTY Moderate   **LENGTH** 4.5 miles
HIGHLIGHTS Lake views, iron ore history, wildlife viewing

THIS TRAIL CIRCLES Honker Lake, which is a winter wildlife refuge, exploring lakeside wetlands, hardwood forest, open lands, and shoreline. The hills aren't too steep or long, making it hikeable by most everyone, despite being 4.5 miles long. First, the trail passes through a wetland, then over Long Creek.

Ahead is an old iron ore pit filled with water that's home to frogs, salamanders, and other aquatic wildlife. Eventually cross long and low Honker Dam, which offers extensive lake views. Pass Goose Islands, then circle around the Nature Station, along with the Woodland Walk. This loop is detailed in the "Nature Station Trails" section on pages 99–100.

■ LAURA FURNACE FORK LOOP

TRAILS USED North–South Trail, Laura Furnace Fork Spur Trail
DIFFICULTY Moderate   **LENGTH** 2.4 miles
HIGHLIGHTS Trail shelter, springs, creek, fields

THIS LOOP TRACES the North–South Trail south to enter the West Fork Laura Furnace Creek watershed. Turn left on the Laura Furnace Fork Spur Trail, which follows the stream, then heads up a spring-fed tributary past narrow fields to reach Laura Furnace Fork trail shelter. Here, two springs provide water for backpackers at the shelter. The yellow-blazed spur trail climbs back into ridgeline hickory-oak woods, passing a hilltop field, then reaches Fords Bay Road. Turn left and follow Fords Bay Road a short piece to complete the loop. Fords Bay Road, Forest Road 170, is 3.7 miles south on Woodlands Trace from the entrance of the Golden Pond Visitor Center. Turn left on Fords Bay Road and follow it for 0.3 mile to the North–South Trail. Begin the loop by heading south on the North–South Trail. You will reach the south end of the Laura Furnace Fork Spur Trail 0.8 mile down the North–South Trail.

MOUNTAIN BIKING LOOPS

WHAT FOLLOWS ARE suggested loop rides in the recreation area. To find the trailhead, simply look at the first trail listed in the "Trails Used" information. If the trail starts at a campground, forest road, or lake access area, the access is in the narrative. "Difficulty" is for average bikers, "Length" is the mileage of the loop, and "Highlights" indicates what is of interest along the way. Some biking loops are on trails only. Other loops use a combination of trails and forest roads. On-trail mountain biking is allowed only north of Golden Pond Visitor Center. Mountain bikes are welcome on paved and gravel roads south of the Golden Pond Visitor Center.

■ BARNETT CREEK/VICKERS CREEK LOOP

TRAILS USED Forest Road 141, Dead Beaver Spring Spur Trail, North–South Trail, FR 339, FR 143
DIFFICULTY Moderate   **LENGTH** 4.4 miles
HIGHLIGHTS Bridge crossings, hills, twisting roads

THIS LOOP STARTS with a climb on FR 143, then steeply descends into Vickers Creek on a twisting dirt road, passing beside a large field before meeting the Dead Beaver Spring Spur Trail. Follow this spur trail a short distance to meet the North–South Trail. The loop follows the North–South Trail south over the ridge back to Barnett Creek Valley. It then travels up rough FR 339, which becomes FR 143 before the loop ends.

To begin the loop, drive north on Woodlands Trace 1.5 miles from the entrance of Golden Pond Visitor Center to FR 141. Turn left on FR 141 and follow it 0.2 mile to intersect FR 143. Park here on the left, beside FR 143. Pedal up and over the hill on FR 141, staying with FR 141 at 0.6 mile where it turns left. Keep downstream along Vickers Creek. The road twists and turns, making for a fun ride. At 2.0 miles, just before FR 141 crosses Vickers Creek, look for a sign that states TO NORTH–SOUTH TRAIL. Veer left off FR 141 onto this path. Soon, reach a trail junction and the North–South Trail. Turn left here and do not cross the wooden bridge over Vickers Creek. Take the North–South Trail south for 1.4 miles.

Emerge onto FR 339. Turn left here, leaving the North–South Trail. Travel up the valley, crossing wet-weather streams and walk beside rock-strewn oak hills. Pass a field as FR 339 becomes FR 141 and complete your loop at 4.4 miles.

■ SUGAR CREEK/IRONTON LOOP

TRAILS USED Forest Road 140, FR 318, FR 139, North–South Trail
DIFFICULTY Moderate to challenging   **LENGTH** 7 miles
HIGHLIGHTS Hills, twisting roads, creek bed crossings

THIS LOOP TAKES you on a roller coaster ride up and down in the Sugar Creek watershed. Leave the Sugar Bay Lake Access Area and climb Ironton Road. Undulate once on the ridgeline, heading for a little-used and rough FR 318. Drop into the North Fork Sugar Creek, where many feeder branches cross the rough road. Climb out of the stream after passing the Sugar Jack Spring trail shelter. Intersect the North–South Trail on gravel County Line Road. Return to Sugar Bay Lake Access via the singletrack North–South Trail.

Hills aplenty will challenge you, and FR 318 is darn near four-wheel-drive territory. The loop leaves the Sugar Bay Lake Access boat ramp. To reach Sugar Bay from the entrance of Golden Pond Visitor Center, take Woodlands Trace north 5.7 miles to FR 140, Ironton Road. Turn left on FR 140 and follow it for 2.1 miles to dead-end at Sugar Bay. Turn left at the lake access to reach the boat ramp parking area.

Leave the lake-access, boat-ramp parking area and return up Ironton Road, passing the North–South Trail that will be your return route. Make a mean climb up the paved portion of Ironton Road before turning left on FR 318 at mile 1.6. This road is barely graveled and very rough. Pass through forest and field, crossing several branches of North Fork Sugar Creek. Look for Sugar Jack trail shelter off to the right at 3.2 miles. Climb past a pond, then down to one more streambed before ascending to reach FR 139, County Line Road. Turn left on FR 139 and intersect the North–South Trail at 4.2 miles.

Descend on FR 139, then leave the forest road after 0.4 mile. Turn left and descend to cross North Fork Sugar Creek on a bridge. Keep south along Sugar Bay, crossing South Fork Sugar Creek. Make one more ascent, then drop to reach Sugar Bay Lake Access after 7.0 miles, completing the loop.

■ NORTH END/NORTH–SOUTH LOOP

TRAILS USED North Paved Trail, North–South Trail
DIFFICULTY Moderate and challenging   **LENGTH** 4.9 miles
HIGHLIGHTS Paved trail, bluff views

THIS LOOP COMBINES some of the easiest and most difficult trail trekking at LBL. Leave the North Welcome Station and warm up on the paved North Paved Trail while heading south to Forest Road 110. After 1.5 miles, turn right on FR 110. After passing under a power line, look right for the white-blazed North–South Trail. Enter a singletrack path on the North–South Trail. Here, the trail dips into hollows and climbs to bluffs overlooking Kentucky Lake, returning to the North Welcome Station after 3.8 challenging miles.

■ CANAL LOOP TRAIL LOOP

TRAILS USED Canal Loop Trail
DIFFICULTY Moderate to difficult   **LENGTH** 10.8 miles
HIGHLIGHTS Views of Lake Barkley and Kentucky Lake

THE CANAL LOOP Trail is the premier mountain biking trail at Land Between The Lakes. It circles the northernmost portion of the LBL peninsula along both lakes. The Lake Barkley side of the loop is generally less hilly. Some rugged and regular ups and downs characterize the last portion of the path. You are likely to see the big barges that ply these waterways on the shoreline portions of these trails. This path is detailed in the "Canal Loop Trails" section of this book on pages 59–63.

PART FOUR

Seeing the Rest of the Park

Road Biking

THE LESSER-TRAVELED YET scenic paved roads of Land Between The Lakes make for great road biking. Although the terrain here is hillier than most would presume, this vertical variation adds a physically challenging dimension to the appealing landscape. The following are suggested road-biking rides, and all are on paved roads. "Road(s) Used" indicates what road(s) the ride follows in the order of their usage; hence, some roads appear twice. "Distance" is the length of the ride. "Highlights" reveals what you will see along the ride. "Facilities" tells what you might find along the way in terms of restrooms and water. A running narrative of the ride follows. Finally, "Access" gives directions to the beginning of the ride.

■ FORT HENRY ROAD RIDE

ROADS USED Fort Henry Road (Forest Road 230), FR 206, FR 172, Woodlands Trace
DISTANCE 35 miles round-trip   **DIFFICULTY** Moderate to difficult
HIGHLIGHTS Homesites, lake views, Cedar Pond, South Bison Range
FACILITIES Water, restrooms, and snacks at South Welcome Station; portable toilets at Cedar Pond Picnic Area

THIS IS ONE of the longer rides at LBL, making a loop from the South Welcome Station, mostly on quiet yet paved forest roads. Start at the South Welcome Station and head west on Fort Henry Road, FR 230. This road is somewhat hilly, and the pavement grain is a little bumpy. Drop into the Panther Creek watershed before turning north onto FR 206. Circle around Dry Fork Bay, passing cemeteries, fields, and old homesites. The road climbs some hills; watch for occasional potholes in the hilly sections. Traverse numerous ridges dividing watersheds to reach North Fork Rushing Creek. Turn right, up FR 172, to reach Woodlands Trace and the state of Kentucky.

Take Woodlands Trace south, shortly reaching Cedar Pond Picnic Area. You are now back in Tennessee. This scenic spot makes for a good resting point: picnic tables are in both sun and shade; portable toilets are located here. A short path circles the pond.

Keep south, undulating over watersheds, and pass The Homeplace and the South Bison Range. Here, buffalo will be grazing in the meadows beside Woodlands Trace. Woodlands Trace continues working in and out of valleys and fields and over wooded hills, returning to the South Welcome Station at 35 miles.

ACCESS This ride starts at the South Welcome Station. From Dover, TN, drive south on US 79 5.0 miles to reach Woodlands Trace. Take Woodlands Trace north 3.4 miles to reach the welcome station.

■ LICK CREEK VALLEY RIDE

ROADS USED Woodlands Trace, Forest Road 165, FR 172
DISTANCE 18 miles round-trip   **DIFFICULTY** Moderate
HIGHLIGHTS Big valleys and fields, homesites, Colson Overlook
FACILITIES Water, restrooms at Golden Pond Visitor Center; portable toilets at Colson Overlook Picnic Area

THE ASCENTS AND descents of this loop ride are more extended than most road combinations in LBL. Start this ride heading south on Woodlands Trace from Golden Pond Visitor Center. Pick up FR 165 as it dips into Elbow Creek. Climb Gordon Hill before enjoying a prolonged descent into Lick Creek. Turn away from Lick Creek near Wranglers Camp. Watch out for horse trailers on FR 165 and equestrians near Wranglers Camp. Look for deer and turkeys in the many roadside fields.

FR 165 turns southwest, climbing over a ridge, then enters lower Laura Furnace Creek. Head up this long valley to reach Woodlands Trace. Just to the south on Woodlands Trace is Cedar Pond Picnic Area, a good resting spot. The ride then turns back north on Woodlands Trace, which straddles the ridgeline dividing the Tennessee River and Cumberland River drainages. Undulate along the ridgeline reaching Colson Overlook Picnic Area, with a far-reaching view of Kentucky Lake to the west. Drop down a long hill into the Turkey Creek drainage. Make one last ascent to reach Golden Pond.

ACCESS This ride starts at the Golden Pond Visitor Center. Golden Pond Visitor Center is centrally located at LBL. It can be reached from the east on I-24 at Exit 65 via US 68/KY 80, from the north on I-24 at Exit 31 via KY 453, from the west by KY 80, and from the south by US 79 and Woodlands Trace.

■ LAKE TO LAKE OUT-AND-BACK RIDE

ROADS USED Old Ferry Road

DISTANCE 22 miles round-trip   **DIFFICULTY** Moderate

HIGHLIGHTS Connects Kentucky Lake to Lake Barkley, quiet road, numerous homesites

FACILITIES Water, restrooms at Birmingham Ferry Campground

TAKE A RIDE through history on this trip. Start at Birmingham Ferry Campground on the shores of Kentucky Lake. Before the rivers were dammed, Between The Rivers residents crossed the Tennessee River on steamboats that landed here. Take Old Ferry Road, leftover from settler days (but paved over since then), and connect to Eddyville Ferry Lake Access, near where folks floated across the Cumberland River. The lesser-traveled Old Ferry Road is mostly in good shape.

Leave the boat-ramp parking area at Birmingham Ferry Campground and cross a small hill. Continue through the campground and begin pedaling up the Pisgah Creek Valley to reach Woodlands Trace. Cross Woodlands Trace. Here, Old Ferry Road traffic decreases. Ridgetop pedaling comes first, before the undulating road enters Mammoth Furnace Creek Valley, where an iron furnace once operated in the 1800s. Beyond here, fields and old homesites border the road. Pass by the large Dickerson Cemetery before dipping toward Lake Barkley. Reach Eddyville Ferry Lake Access, which has a boat ramp and paved auto turnaround at 11.0 miles. Turn around on your bike and backtrack through this northeastern tip of LBL, recrossing Woodlands Trace and returning to Birmingham Ferry Campground.

ACCESS From the North Welcome Station, take Woodlands Trace south 5.3 miles to paved Forest Road 117, Old Ferry Road. Turn right on Old Ferry Road and follow it 3.5 miles to dead-end at the campground. Park at the very far end of the campground near the boat ramp.

■ SILVER TRAIL RIDE

ROADS USED Woodlands Trace, Mulberry Flats Road, Forest Road 134, Silver Trail Road

DISTANCE 11 miles round-trip   **DIFFICULTY** Easy to moderate

HIGHLIGHTS Nature Station, Hematite Lake, Center Furnace Ruins

FACILITIES Water, restrooms at Nature Station

THIS RIDE IS less hilly than most at LBL. However, don't expect completely level terrain here. This ride leaves southbound on Woodlands Trace, then heads east on Mulberry Flats Road. Descend to reach Hematite Lake and Center Furnace, where ore was smelted into iron. Nearby, Hematite Lake Picnic Area makes a good stopping point. You are now in the Nature Station recreation complex, which offers hiking trails, wildlife observation, and more. Leave this area on the old Silver Trail Road and return to your starting point along Woodlands Trace.

Begin the ride by heading south on Woodlands Trace. The road has some ups and downs as it courses into the upper end of the Long Creek Valley above Barnes Hollow. Reach Mulberry Flats Road at mile 2.4. Turn left on Mulberry Flats Road, FR 135. Fields dotted with trees along the roadside are improved wild turkey habitat. The road makes a nearly imperceptible downgrade. At 6.4 miles, turn left on FR 134, which descends to Hematite Lake and Center Furnace ruins. The stone and brick furnace ruins are visible from the road. Hematite Lake Picnic Area is to your left. Just ahead, to your right, is the Nature Station. Save your visit for when you have plenty of time.

At mile 7.7, turn left on Silver Trail Road. Ascend along this historic road. Back when Center Furnace was operating, legend has it that workers were paid in silver and the company pay wagon, loaded with silver, took this road to the furnace to pay the workers. Silver Trail Road works its way onto a ridgeline to meet Woodlands Trace at 11.0 miles.

ACCESS   This ride starts at the intersection of Woodlands Trace and Silver Trail Road. From the entrance of Golden Pond Visitor Center, take Woodlands Trace north 9.4 miles to Silver Trail Road. A small gravel parking area is on the left just after this turn. Begin the ride by heading south on Woodlands Trace.

■ WOODLANDS TRACE ONE-WAY RIDE

ROADS USED Woodlands Trace
DISTANCE 40 miles one-way   **DIFFICULTY** Moderate to difficult
HIGHLIGHTS Travels from one end of LBL to the other, South Bison Range, The Homeplace, Golden Pond Visitor Center
FACILITIES Water, restrooms at North Welcome Station, Golden Pond Visitor Center, South Welcome Station; portable toilets at picnic areas

THIS IS THE premier long-distance ride at LBL. Woodlands Trace sees its share of auto traffic, but not too much, especially during the week. The only time I wouldn't do this ride is on holiday weekends. Facilities are located at either end of the ride. Golden Pond Visitor Center lies in the middle. Picnic areas are scattered along the ride, making for frequent potential stopping points. In the north, Woodlands Trace mostly follows the backbone of the ridge dividing the Tennessee River and Cumberland River watersheds. It has some hills but not like the second half of the road, which repetitively dips into creeks and climbs over the ridges dividing the creeks. The climbs are never overly long, but they do come regularly.

Leave the North Welcome Station and shortly pass Star Camp Picnic Area. Woodlands Trace stays along the Tennessee Divide, curving past woods and fields. Pass Jenny Ridge Picnic Area just before reaching Golden Pond Visitor Center, the halfway point.

Keep south past the visitor center. Woodlands Trace changes character, heading deeper into creeks flowing west from the divide and over ridgelines separating the creeks. Pass Colson Overlook Picnic Area, then, once into Tennessee, Cedar Pond Picnic Area. Woodlands Trace switches over to the east side of the recreation area, passing the South Bison Range, where the buffalo roam. The road climbs in and out of creeks flowing east. Reach the South Welcome Station and end the ride. Avid, in-shape bikers will turn around and head back. But most riders will have arranged a shuttle ride or left a car here.

ACCESS This ride starts at the North Welcome Station. From Exit 31 on I-24 near Lake City, head south on KY 453 for 7.0 miles, intersecting Woodlands Trace along the way to reach the North Welcome Station.

Scenic Drives

LAND BETWEEN THE Lakes offers auto tourists many driving options, from the paved Trace to rough back roads requiring four-wheel drive. The following scenic drives can be made in a passenger car. Gravel roads are part of some drives. LBL roads are numbered. Those starting with a "1" or "2" are generally passable in a passenger car. Anything goes on a road starting with the number "3." Don't even think about going on a road that starts with "4." There are some exceptions to the numbering system, especially roads leading to cemeteries. The back roads of LBL beckon exploration, but stay within the limits of your vehicle. Tow trucks can be expensive. A word to the wise: before you start on a forest drive, get an LBL Legal Roads Map at the North Welcome Station, South Welcome Station, or Golden Pond Visitor Center. It shows all legal roads in LBL and details the many cemeteries. This way, if you decide to break off on your own, you can keep apprised of your position.

■ WOODLANDS TRACE SCENIC DRIVE

TYPE Paved drive   **LENGTH** 40 miles one way
HIGHLIGHTS Great Western Iron Furnace, The Homeplace, Buffalo Range, Elk & Bison Prairie,
Colson Overlook   **AMENITIES** Welcome stations, visitor center, picnic areas

THE WOODLANDS TRACE is the master road of Land Between The Lakes, the
backbone of the road system here. This two-lane paved road extends the length of the
peninsula from US 79 near Dover in the south to the canal linking Lake Barkley and
Kentucky Lake in the north. It runs north to south, roughly parallel to the lakes. Along
the way, it passes through scenery typical of the LBL: forests, fields, hickory-oak ridges,
and rocky streambeds beneath hardwood hollows.

Leave the South Welcome Station and travel north. The undulating character
of this road is soon evident. Much of the road travels along the ridgeline dividing
the Tennessee and Cumberland River drainages. However, the road starts cours-
ing through several watersheds. Span Barrett Creek near the former community of
Tharpe. Ahead on Woodlands Trace is a still-standing historic structure—the Great

Great Western Iron Furnace

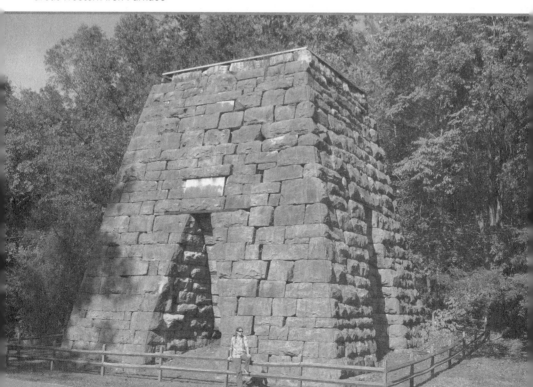

Western Iron Furnace. This limestone stack was used in the process of turning ore into iron. The South Bison Range lies just to the north. Buffalo have been restored to this land where they ranged more than two centuries ago. The next potential stop is The Homeplace, a living farm offering live demonstrations of life Between The Rivers as it was back in the mid-1800s.

Shortly, enter the Bluegrass State, just after passing scenic Cedar Pond. Make sure to stop at Colson Overlook to view Kentucky Lake to the west. Woodlands Trace leads to Golden Pond Visitor Center, which offers information and services. Consider a side trip to the Elk & Bison Prairie, where the large animals roam a restored prairie looking much as it did in presettler days. Woodlands Trace then continues along the Tennessee Divide, winding past field and forest in the LBL's northern end before arriving at the North Welcome Station.

ACCESS From Dover, TN, head south on US 79 5.0 miles to access Woodlands Trace. Turn right on Woodlands Trace and drive north 3.4 miles to reach the South Welcome Station on your right. This scenic drive starts at the South Welcome Station.

■ NORTH FIGURE-EIGHT SCENIC DRIVE

TYPE Mostly paved   **LENGTH** 27 miles round-trip
HIGHLIGHTS Bluff-top views of Kentucky Lake, homesites, historical markers
AMENITIES North Welcome Station, Star Camp Picnic Area

THIS SCENIC DRIVE route actually covers an LBL-designated scenic drive and then some. Start at the North Welcome Center and head north to the edge of LBL and take Kentucky Lake Scenic Drive, with breathtaking views of Kentucky Lake, then return to Woodlands Trace. Head south on Woodlands Trace and take Birmingham Ferry Road to the little-visited northeastern section of LBL, returning via Brandon Chapel Road. Most of the road is paved, but Brandon Chapel does have two small creek crossings that should be passable by all cars nearly all year long.

Leave the North Welcome Station and join Woodlands Trace heading northbound. Turn left onto Kentucky Lake Scenic Drive. Curve past the canal connecting Kentucky Lake and Lake Barkley, which together form one of the largest man-made bodies of water in the world. The road then turns south and over some bluffs along Kentucky Lake. Pullovers lead to the edge of these bluffs and expansive views of Kentucky Lake.

Emerge onto Woodlands Trace and turn right, heading south. Shortly, pass Star Camp Picnic Area, a fine place for a barbecue or a sandwich. Woodlands Trace becomes curvy amid pine trees. Ahead, turn left on paved Old Ferry Road, Forest Road 117. This is one of the quietest paved roads in the recreation area. Pass the Mammoth Furnace historical marker, then turn left onto FR 124 just as you reach the large and open Dickerson Cemetery.

FR 124 is gravel. Stay with it just a short distance and veer left on FR 112. Undulate through the hills around Carmack Creek. The road fords Carmack Creek, which is normally dry. Pass fields and woods, making a last ford of Demumbers Creek, another often-dry stream. Ahead is the site of Paradise Christian Church. Reach Woodlands Trace at another historical marker, this one about Kentucky governor Keen Johnson. Return north on Woodlands Trace to North Welcome Station.

ACCESS   From Exit 31 on I-24 near Lake City, head south on KY 453 for 7.0 miles. KY 453 becomes Woodlands Trace once it enters Land Between The Lakes National Recreation Area. The North Welcome Station will be on your right.

■ SOUTH LOOP FOREST DRIVE

TYPE Mostly paved with some gravel   **LENGTH** 35 miles round-trip
HIGHLIGHTS Kentucky Lake and Lake Barkley bay views, homesites
AMENITIES South Welcome Station, Neville Bay Lake Access

IF YOU ARE looking for a forest drive in the wooded hinterlands of LBL, this is it. This loop drive travels lesser-used roads of LBL's Tennessee side. Most of the roads are paved, but there are some gravel roads and two creek fords that are passable about 95% of the time by passenger cars. The loop leaves South Welcome Station and travels west on Fort Henry Road, then turns north along Kentucky Lake where bay views await. It keeps north, crossing into Kentucky before turning south on a gravel road that sees little traffic. Then it returns to Tennessee, enjoying bay views of Lake Barkley before intersecting Woodlands Trace north of the South Welcome Station. Head south on Woodlands Trace to complete the loop.

Begin the scenic drive on Fort Henry Road, Forest Road 230, which leaves west from the South Welcome Station. This paved road heads toward Kentucky Lake, veering right on paved FR 206 at 4.0 miles. Reach open fields and hilltop forests while passing bays. Stay with FR 206 as it zigzags ever north to reach FR 172 at 21.0 miles near Rushing Creek Campground. Turn right on paved FR 172 to reach Woodlands Trace and Kentucky. Cross Woodlands Trace and pick up paved FR 165. Watch for horses in this area, as many equestrians ride out from Wranglers Campground.

Leave paved FR 165 after a concrete ford of an unnamed stream and turn right onto gravel FR 174. Immediately after this turn, FR 174 fords Laura Furnace Creek on a concrete crossing. Laura Furnace Creek doesn't even flow at this point much of the year, so the crossing is nearly always doable. FR 174 oozes solitude as it crisscrosses ridges between wide bottomlands. A great lake view can be had when the road crosses Prior Bay. The road enters Tennessee without fanfare, then briefly veers left on FR 204, and then veers right on FR 214 past numerous homesites. Views open again when passing Neville Bay Lake Access. Soon, reach Woodlands Trace and head south to the South Welcome Station.

ACCESS From Dover, TN, head south on US 79 for 5.0 miles to access Woodlands Trace. Turn right on Woodlands Trace and drive north for 3.4 miles to reach the South Welcome Station on your right. This scenic drive starts at the South Welcome Station.

Picnic Areas

THE NATIONAL RECREATION area has several designated picnic areas for visitors to enjoy. Recreation opportunities are near all picnic areas, enabling you to work off those hamburgers and hot dogs. The following is a list of those picnic areas, along with suggested area activities. Note that other areas such as North Welcome Station, South Welcome Station, and Golden Pond Visitor Center also have picnicking spots.

SOUTH BISON RANGE

THE SOUTH BISON Range Picnic Area is located on Woodlands Trace across from LBL's South Bison Range, a fenced area where the buffalo roam. A massive, beautiful white oak tree fronts the old homesite turned picnic area. Large maples shade the five moderately used picnic tables situated on a grassy lawn. Hilly woods rise away from an intermittent streambed behind the lawn. Stand-up grills are available for cooking. Two portable toilets are located nearby.

Watching for buffalo is a natural pastime here. A field stretches out before picnickers. If you want to hike, the Model Loop Trail makes a 7.5-mile circuit around the South Bison Range and along the Tennessee Ridge. It starts a half mile north at The Homeplace trailhead. A shorter loop cuts across the South Bison Range. After the shortcut, you can go left or right along the South Bison Range fence. This shortcut is 0.2 mile north of the picnic area, on the west side of Woodlands Trace. Look for the wooden bridge spanning Prior Creek. An informative walk would include a tour of The Homeplace, located just north on Woodlands Trace. More picnic tables are located at

The Homeplace trailhead. To reach the trailhead, turn right into The Homeplace, then immediately turn left before you cross Prior Creek and follow the gravel road a short distance to the gravel parking area. The picnic tables are next to Prior Creek.

ACCESS From the South Welcome Station, head north on Woodlands Trace for 10.1 miles to the picnic area, on your right.

CEDAR POND

CEDAR POND PICNIC Area is located on Woodlands Trace just south of the Tennessee–Kentucky state line. The small impoundment is ringed in cedar trees mixed with hardwoods. Five picnic tables are situated in two locations. Two tables are beneath a tall and shady cedar grove. The other three tables lie beneath tall pines in a mix of sun and shade. Stand-up grills are available for cooking. Portable toilets and trash receptacles are located at the site too.

Cedar Pond, a relic from a former farm, is especially scenic in fall when the autumn colors reflect off the still pond, contrasting with blue skies and green cedars.

Cedar Pond Picnic Area

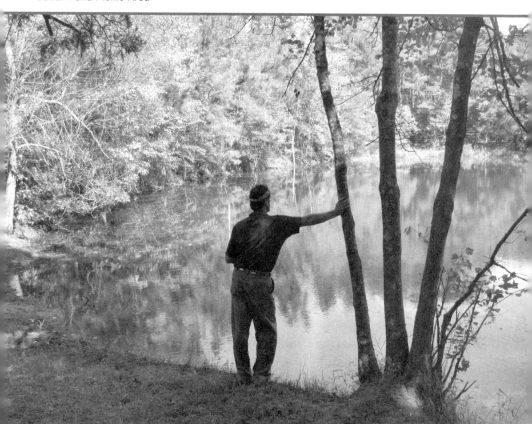

A short gravel trail leads across the dam and around the little lake. Two boardwalks cross the branches that feed Cedar Pond, where turtles will be sunning on logs. Anglers use this path to access fishing points. The South Bison Range and The Homeplace are a few miles south of Cedar Pond.

ACCESS From the South Welcome Station, head north on Woodlands Trace for 12.7 miles to the picnic area, on your right, just before the Tennessee–Kentucky state line.

COLSON OVERLOOK

COLSON OVERLOOK PICNIC AREA stands beside Woodlands Trace a few miles north of the Tennessee state line. From this high point, picnickers can look miles west to Kentucky Lake, though the trees have grown up as of late. A lone chestnut oak tree shades two picnic tables near the entrance. A second set of tables lies beneath a stand of tall pines, offering a mix of sun and shade. Stand-up grills are located at each area for cooking. An accessible vault toilet and a trash receptacle are beside the gravel parking area. An equestrian picnic area is located just down the hill from the main picnic area. This level, shaded spot overlooks a small pond and has a hitching post for horses.

Hikers can use an access trail that leads east down the steep hill to reach the North–South Trail. In times past, I have walked south on the North–South Trail to Forest Road 170, taken FR 170 to Woodlands Trace, and then walked north on Woodlands Trace back to Colson for a little leg-stretching loop. More ambitious hikers can tack on the 2.4-mile Laura Furnace Fork Loop, which keeps south on the North–South Trail at FR 170 (See "Suggested Loops," page 143). More developed activities are ongoing at Golden Pond Visitor Center, which is just a few miles north of here.

ACCESS From the entrance to the Golden Pond Visitor Center, drive south on Woodlands Trace for 3.4 miles to the picnic area, on your left.

HEMATITE LAKE

HEMATITE LAKE PICNIC AREA is located amid the Nature Station recreation complex. If you are looking for a picnic locale with plenty to do nearby, Hematite Lake is for you. The picnic area is set in a flat beside Long Creek, which at this point serves as the outflow for Hematite Lake. Hardwoods shade the initial few sites, which are backed up against a hill. Each site has a picnic table and fire grate. The ruins of Center Furnace are visible in the distance. A gravel road passes these first sites and continues to the Hematite Lake dam. Two more sites and accessible vault toilets are located up here. The lake waters flowing over the dam serenade picnickers on this upper end. A final set of three picnic tables overlooks the dam on the beginning of the Hematite Lake Trail.

Most activities are within walking distance of the picnic area. Walking is an activity unto itself here, as the 2.2-mile Hematite Lake Trail circles the waterfowl-attracting impoundment. The 0.3-mile Center Furnace Trail starts around the corner, as does the 0.2-mile Long Creek Trail. The 1.0-mile Woodland Walk starts at the Nature Station, an environmental education area where visitors can see and enjoy wildlife.

Others will be seen bank fishing Long Creek, which flows directly past the picnic area. Just upstream, anglers can either bank fish Hematite Lake or launch their boats. Hematite is a "no gas motors" lake, offering a peaceful angling experience, as well as paddling and wildlife watching from your canoe.

ACCESS   From the entrance of Golden Pond Visitor Center, head north on Woodlands Trace for 7.0 miles to Mulberry Flats Road, Forest Road 135. Turn right on Mulberry Flats Road and follow it for 4.0 miles to FR 134. Turn left on FR 134 and follow it for a mile to the picnic area on your left just before Center Furnace ruins.

JENNY RIDGE

JENNY RIDGE STANDS on a hill beside Woodlands Trace just north of Golden Pond Visitor Center. Just the right number of oaks shade the grassy lawn, where 10 picnic tables and grills await your arrival. Spots are nearly always available at this lesser-used area. The hill commands a view of Woodlands Trace, yet having to carry the goodies a short distance up some steps to the sites seems to dissuade most picnickers. Maybe they could use a "jenny," or mule, to carry their supplies. Legend has it this place was named for a mule that was lost around here. A second story has it that a man with the last name of Jenny strung a telegraph line past here.

You won't need to ride a mule to access the portable toilet, conveniently located at the picnic parking area. If you want to ride your mountain bike or go for a little hike, the North–South Trail is just 0.2 mile down the yellow-blazed Jenny Ridge Spur Trail, which leaves from the parking area. This section of the North–South Trail is open to bikes. Northbound trail trekkers will head into Barnett Creek Valley. Most visitors to Jenny Ridge will be planning their trip to, or reflecting on their trip from, the Elk & Bison Prairie located just across Woodlands Trace. This self-guided auto tour travels through a restored prairie, which is authentic even down to the native grasses. The area is designed to look as it did 200 years ago, when elk and bison freely roamed the barrens of western Kentucky.

ACCESS   From the entrance of Golden Pond Visitor Center, head north on Woodlands Trace 0.8 mile to reach Jenny Ridge on your left.

STAR CAMP

STAR CAMP PICNIC Area is a pleasing stopover. Situated off Woodlands Trace, the area looks like a good place to break in the midst of an LBL adventure. The paved road enters a loop that winds through a gently rolling hill dotted with big shade trees. Underneath is a grassy lawn. Five concrete picnic tables are spread far and wide among the trees. A grill accompanies each picnic table. Accessible vault toilets serve visitors. Being a little off Woodlands Trace adds solitude.

One theory holds that this picnic area got its name from the former Star Lime Works. This company was in the business of extracting mineral lime. Lime is obtained by heating limestone until it crumbles to powder. Lime is used in fertilizer and for making cement.

Star Camp Picnic Area is great for a cookout. Bring some food here and relax, watching the sun move the shadows across the grass. The Pisgah Point Lake Access Area is just a short way down Forest Road 111. Here, you can look out on Kentucky Lake and maybe do a little bank fishing. The North–South Trail crosses FR 111 near the lake. Other trails are north of here. A good idea might be a rustic forest drive down Brandon Chapel Road, which leaves just across Woodlands Trace. Return via paved Old Ferry Road. See "North Figure-Eight Scenic Drive," pages 152–153.

ACCESS From the North Welcome Station, drive south on Woodlands Trace 3.1 miles to paved FR 111. Turn right and reach the Star Camp Picnic Area on your right.

PART FIVE

• Places •
to Lay Your Head

Camping

CAMPING AT LBL can range from backpacking overnight on a remote trail to enjoying full hookups at a developed campground. Land Between The Lakes has several developed campgrounds with varied facilities. Campers can also overnight it at most lesser-developed lake access areas, beside most backwoods roads, deep in the woods, or on an undeveloped shoreline. However, if you decide to camp somewhere other than a fee campground *you must purchase a backcountry camping permit.* Once purchased, this backcountry permit is good for a year from the date of purchase, no matter if you stay one night or many more at LBL. A three-day permit is also available for purchase. *Note:* each person 18 years old and older who backcountry camps is required to purchase a backcountry camping permit.

There are exceptions. Backpackers hiking and camping overnight on the North–South Trail, Canal Loop Trails, or Fort Henry Trails, moving from campsite to campsite each day, are not required to purchase the backcountry camping permit but are required to obtain a Free Backpacking Permit. Additionally, if you are staying in a fee campground, you do not need to buy a backcountry permit in addition to paying the fee at that campground.

Camping is permitted anywhere at LBL except the following:

1. within cemetery boundaries;
2. within 200 yards of Woodlands Trace or other major roads as posted;
3. within the Environmental Education Area;
4. other sites as posted.

Campers can camp at one area a maximum of 14 consecutive days in backcountry locations, 21 days at developed, fee campgrounds.

Campgrounds

■ BIRMINGHAM FERRY/SMITH BAY

NEAREST TOWN Grand Rivers, KY   **OPEN** Year-round   **INDIVIDUAL SITES** Birmingham Ferry 29, Smith Bay 16   **EACH SITE** Picnic table, fire grate   **SITE ASSIGNMENT** First come, first served; no reservations   **REGISTRATION** On site   **FACILITIES** Vault toilets   **FEE** Yes, backcountry camping permit required for each camper 18 and over

BIRMINGHAM FERRY CAMPGROUND is moderately sized, rustic, and has many lakeside campsites. Just a ridge over to the south is the Smith Bay Campground. No matter which one of the two you choose, all sorts of water-recreation opportunities are at hand on Kentucky Lake. Trails for mountain bikers, open to hikers as well, are just a pedal away.

Old Ferry Road ends near Kentucky Lake and enters the Birmingham Ferry Campground. The first couple of sites in the loop are wide open and away from the lake, about 100 feet from the water. A few trees begin to shade some of the later sites, then the loop turns left toward the water, where seven large, somewhat open sites lie directly on Kentucky Lake.

A road continues away from the water. Climb a small ridge on this road and dip again to the lake, this time into Pisgah Bay. Drop to the water and reach two isolated sites directly on the bay. Boaters claim these sites early. Pass the boat ramp and boater parking area, then reach an unlikely loop on an ultrasteep hill. Two sites standing on a bluff offer great views, but make sure to tie yourself in or you might take a tumble. These sites have expansive water vistas, though they are not suitable for kids. Swing around and climb higher on the hill to a couple more sites on a more reasonable slope where sites have been leveled.

Head over to Smith Ridge Campground before you make your final campsite decision. Pass campsite 16, all by itself on the water, to reach the boat launch, then enter the main campground. It is very open, but sites usually have a shade tree or two to keep the sun at bay. Pass a string of seven lakeside sites then turn away from the water. These sites up the hill are better shaded and offer a view of Smith Bay. This campground, like Birmingham Ferry, has convenient vault toilets and a water spigot.

Water recreation is immediate from either campground. Boating, fishing, and swimming are likely choices. If the winds are high on Kentucky Lake, both Smith Bay and Pisgah Bay are large enough to offer plenty of fishing. The reason I enjoy these areas is the land-based recreation. The North–South Trail crosses Old Ferry Road just a half mile from Birmingham Ferry. This section of the North–South Trail is open to hikers and mountain bikers. You can pedal directly from the campground. Head south toward Hatchery Hollow and use forest roads to complete a loop. If heading north, you will come to a side trail reaching Nightriders Spring, then a paved hike/bike trail that makes a loop out of Hillman Ferry Campground.

Farther north are the Canal Loop Trails. A series of connector trails makes loop routes possible here, ranging from a mile to ten or more. Wear yourself out, but first get a trail map at the North Welcome Center to know where you are going.

ACCESS From the North Welcome Station, take Woodlands Trace south 5.3 miles to paved Forest Road 117, Old Ferry Road. Turn right on Old Ferry Road and follow it 3.5 miles to dead-end at the campground.

■ CRAVENS BAY

NEAREST TOWN Grand Rivers, KY OPEN Year-round INDIVIDUAL SITES 31 EACH SITE Picnic table, fire grate, some have tent pads SITE ASSIGNMENT First come, first served; no reservations REGISTRATION Self-registration, on site FACILITIES Water spigot, flush toilets FEE Yes

CRAVENS BAY IS off the beaten path at LBL. Folks seeking solitude come here to relax at a scenic lakeside camp that attracts mostly campers in RVs and trailers. A campground host allows for an easier and safer stay, making this quiet spot even more desirable.

Enter the lower Cravens Creek Valley. Cravens Bay, part of Lake Barkley, appears on your right. At the campground, pass the wide and convenient boat ramp with its large gravel parking area. A courtesy dock floats beside the ramp. On your left are picnic sites carved into the side of the hill. Wide steps lead up to campground restrooms that have flush toilets from March through November, but no showers. Ahead is the campground. Three campsites stand on the hill to the left. The campground host's site fronts the main campground loop. The loop circles a flat beside the lake and has 15 sites beside Cravens Bay. These sites have been leveled and are shaded by a line of trees. RVs and pop-up campers like to set up here.

You may think this loop is the end of the campground, but hold on. A gravel road runs alongside Cravens Bay away from the main loop. Soon, a couple more sites are set in a small flat beside the shore. The gravel road continues a half mile farther to reach a second loop. Five large sites are set on a shaded hill away from the lake. The gravel road continues to a grassy field broken by a few hackberry and maple trees. A steep boat ramp lies at the end of the loop. Six sites, better suited for tent campers, overlook Lake Barkley from a hill. Most have ample shade. This "Mystery Loop" is less popular but would be great for family campers who want room to roam and have a little fun without getting in their neighbor's hair. Portable toilets serve this isolated area.

Recreation at Cravens Bay is centered on the water. Boating, fishing, and swimming are your choices. Other recreation opportunities require a bit of a drive. That is why you see many self-contained big rigs here. They set up, lay up, and relax. And if that is on your agenda, then make Cravens Bay your LBL headquarters and leave the running around to others.

ACCESS From the North Welcome Station, take Woodlands Trace south 5.3 miles to paved Forest Road 117, Old Ferry Road. Turn left on Old Ferry Road and follow it 1.4 miles to paved FR 118. Turn right on FR 118 and follow it 2.9 miles to dead-end at the campground.

■ ENERGY LAKE

NEAREST TOWN Canton, KY **OPEN** March–October **INDIVIDUAL SITES** 48 total, 41 with electricity **EACH SITE** Picnic table, fire grate, some have tent pads **SITE ASSIGNMENT** First come, first served and by reservation; 800-525-7077, or online at **landbetweenthelakes.us /reservations** **REGISTRATION** At campground entrance station **FACILITIES** Hot showers, flush toilets, telephone, ice machine, cabins (sleep 4–6), dump station **FEE** Yes

ENERGY LAKE IS an ideal example of enhancing natural resources to create a better recreation area. Start with a rolling shoreline on a scenic body of water. Integrate a just-the-right-size campground into the landscape, add a few amenities such as electricity and hot showers, and hold on to that rustic feel. What you end up with is a complete camping package.

Cross the dam that separates Energy Lake from Lake Barkley and enter the campground. Pass the entrance station and climb a hill to Area A. The 12 sites are attractively set on a high peninsula. The sites are leveled with landscaping timbers. Seven of the sites overlook the lake, which is 60 feet below, offering a watery panorama. The camping pads are large and well spaced but don't have too much of an understory. A fully equipped bathhouse lies in the center of Area A, as on all four loops. It also has two of the unusual shelter houses. Tent campers can use these three-sided shelters, with a picnic table inside, during rainy times to cook or just hang out, which can help a lot when the weather is bad. However, you can't just set your gear up and sleep in here. So, keep your bedding in your tent.

There will be a mix of RVs and tents at Energy Lake, but Area B, with only two electric sites, is the domain of the canvas set. This loop, the only one away from the lake, heads higher up the hill. The sites are spacious here beneath hickory-oak woodland. Two shelter houses and two water spigots make camping life a little more comfortable.

Pass the day-use area, which is down a steep road leading to a grassy flat. A swim beach and play area, with a court, small ball field, and a horseshoe pit are here. Area C is an unusual loop. Drop down a hill, passing some large sites, and come to a lakeside site. The loop road then makes a figure eight, with three prime lakeside sites. Turn away from the lake, where four more commendable campsites are located. Area D is a little down the main campground road. The road drops so steeply that you might think an elevator would better serve the tiered campsites beside the road. Make no mistake, these sites are level and attractive. The road is scary, though. A couple of shelter houses are here too. Also, more lake-view sites are here, though most are away from the water.

All campsites can be reserved. If you want to start relaxing early, phone in that reservation, then cruise on to Energy Lake. I recommend reservations on summer weekends. Bring your boat to enjoy the 370-acre, no-wake impoundment or nearby Lake Barkley, which is just across the dam road over which you drove. If you don't have a boat, rent a canoe here. Many folks paddle for fun or cast their rod for crappie, catfish, or bass. Energy Dam Lake Access has a fishing pier for boatless anglers. Two hiking trails totaling more than 6 miles can be accessed right from your campsite. They wind and roll all over this hilly country, making two loops. A small trail map is included on the campground map.

The Nature Station is nearby. It offers environmental education in an attractive setting. The Learning Center has exhibits on the wildlife of Land Between The Lakes. The Backyard has animals that have been taken in by the Nature Station, along with plants native to this region. There are also aquatic creatures in the turtle and fish ponds. You can see a bald eagle, owls, bobcats, coyotes, deer, and more. Kids can really have a good time, and the adults might learn a thing or two themselves. Another set of trails emanates from the Nature Station. The Center Furnace Trail checks out the remnants of a great iron furnace and the iron industry of this area. The Hematite and Honker Trails circle small lakes, offering possibilities of seeing waterfowl. You can also rent canoes to paddle Honker Lake. Energy Lake is a good base camp for active campers at LBL.

ACCESS   From the North Welcome Station, take Woodlands Trace south 9.0 miles to Forest Road 133, Silver Trail Road. Turn left on Silver Trail Road and follow it 3.0 miles to FR 134. Turn right on FR 134 and follow it 4.5 miles to the campground, on your right.

■ FENTON

NEAREST TOWN Aurora, KY   **OPEN** Year-round   **INDIVIDUAL SITES** 29 total, 11 with electricity   **EACH SITE** Picnic table, fire grate   **SITE ASSIGNMENT** First come, first served   **REGISTRATION** Self-registration, on site   **FACILITIES** Water spigot, accessible vault toilets   **FEE** Yes

FENTON CAMPGROUND IS on the site of the old Fenton community. Located adjacent to US 68/KY 80 beside Kentucky Lake, this campground is also a special events area. The wide field next to the campground is used for arts and crafts fairs, fishing tournaments, and family reunions. Turn off US 68/KY 80 and enter Fenton. To your right is a row of 12 open sites backed against a line of sycamore and sweet gum trees. Being on the north side of these trees does provide some shade, but the sites themselves are out in the open with no privacy from one another. The sites have been graveled, and it gives them a parking lot–like appearance. A row of pine trees slightly screens them from the road, but not from road noise. Vault toilets are near these sites.

A long rock jetty protects the three-wide boat ramp from the bulk of Kentucky Lake. A courtesy dock allows easy entry and exit for boaters. The rock jetty also serves as a bank-fishing venue. Across from the jetty are four more campsites directly on the

Picnic Shelter at Fenton

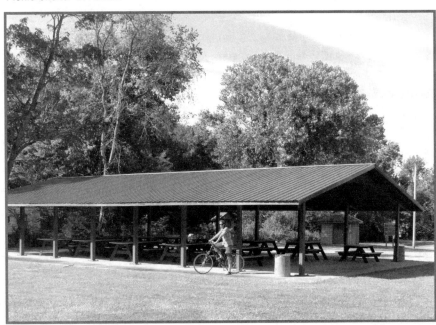

water. The old US 68/KY 80 route is used to access these sites that overlook the boat ramp. They are small and close to the current US 68/KY 80 route, but they stay busy.

The 11 electricity-supplied sites are away from the highway. Head away from old US 68/KY 80 to reach the first few sites, which are set beneath trees shading a rocky streambed. A concrete ford crosses the streambed, which is usually dry, to the rest of the campsites. These sites are banked against a tree-covered hill. Some are shaded, some are open to the sun. Campsite privacy is limited here too. Small wooden foot-bridges span the streambed to access the special-events field. Vault toilets are here too.

Fenton is a lesser-used campground, except during special events. A large picnic pavilion is used during special events and by large groups. Boaters who want convenient access to the boat ramp are the primary users. General recreationalists exploring LBL seek quieter camping areas. This is the western trailhead for the Central Hardwoods Scenic Trail, popular with bicyclers.

ACCESS   From the entrance of the Golden Pond Visitor Center, drive south on Woodlands Trace a quarter mile to Golden Pond Road. Turn left on Golden Pond Road and follow it 0.3 mile to US 68/KY 80. Turn left, heading west, and follow US 68/KY 80 2.5 miles to the campground, on your left, just before the bridge over Kentucky Lake.

■ GATLIN POINT

NEAREST TOWN Dover, TN   **OPEN** Year-round   **INDIVIDUAL SITES** 19   **EACH SITE** Picnic table, fire grate   **SITE ASSIGNMENT** First come, first served; no reservations   **REGISTRATION** Self-registration, on site   **FACILITIES** Water spigot, courtesy dock, accessible vault toilets   **FEE** Yes

THIS IS A boater's campground. Gatlin Point Campground overlooks two lakes, Bards Lake and Lake Barkley. However, only a low dam over which a paved road runs separates these lakes. A north-facing wooded hill is the setting for this campground. Keep forward on the access road and turn left into the campground just before reaching the dam. Three campsites are located near the lake and are shaded by the afternoon sun. Another site is located in the open, in a grassy area overlooking the lake. It offers good views but no privacy. More sites are up the hill and are shaded by oaks of varying ages, along with a few cedars. A grassy understory complements the sites, which are a little close together.

More secluded sites are located away from the lake. Of special note is campsite 19, tucked away near an intermittent stream. Two reliable water spigots are provided for the campground, as are vault toilets.

Three hundred twenty–acre Bards Lake is divided from Lake Barkley by the dam. This is a no-wake lake with a primitive gravel launch at the low point of the campground. Anglers in smaller boats will enjoy the scenery and maybe a few fish on the end of the line. The grassy locale of Brandon Spring Group Center is visible across Bards Lake. A bona fide concrete launch is located on the far side of the dam, allowing motorboat access to Lake Barkley. At this point, Lake Barkley resembles a long strand of water broken by several small, ribbon-like islands. Gated fire roads spur out from the campground and could serve as informal trails if you wanted to stretch your legs.

ACCESS From the South Welcome Station, take Woodlands Trace north 0.9 mile to Forest Road 227. Turn right on FR 227 and follow it 2.0 miles. Veer left on FR 229 and follow it 1.5 miles, and the campground will be on your left.

■ HILLMAN FERRY

NEAREST TOWN Grand Rivers, KY **OPEN** March–November **INDIVIDUAL SITES** 100 basic sites; 45 electric; 157 electric and water; 72 electric, water, and sewer **EACH SITE** Picnic table, fire grate; some have lantern posts; others varying combination of electric, water, and sewer **SITE ASSIGNMENT** First come, first served and by reservation; 800-525-7077, or online at **landbetweenthelakes.us/reservations** **REGISTRATION** At campground gatehouse **FACILITIES** Hot showers, water spigots, camp store, laundry **FEE** Yes, rates rise with varying combinations of electric, water, and sewer at each site

HILLMAN FERRY IS the big campground in the northern end of Land Between The Lakes. Piney Campground is the big one in the south. Hillman Ferry has 376 campsites! It takes a few miles of driving to see them all. Determined campers will find a site at this campground that offers something for nearly everyone.

Pass the campground gatehouse, operated by friendly folks who are here to help. Turn right and enter Area A. It is newer and offers 82 mostly shaded campsites. Area A is open April–August. The first 20 sites offer electricity and water and are very popular. The next set has basic, leveled sites beneath hardwoods. More sites surround a modern bathhouse. Beyond the bathhouse are many campsites overlooking a cove of Kentucky Lake. These lakeside sites are scenic, but will not be quiet during summer, as they look out on the campground's swim beach and volleyball court. These sites, though, would be good for families with children. A boat ramp with a courtesy dock is also in this cove. The campground road continues around the cove and climbs a hill. These hilltop sites have been renovated and offer great lake views but require

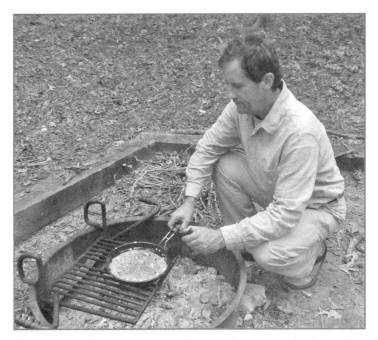

The author cooks pancakes over the fire while camped at Hillman Ferry Campground.

campers to haul their gear up or down to the campsite. Boaters like them because they can pull their boats to the shoreline adjacent to the lower campsites.

Area B, with 68 sites, is open from May through September. The spur roads overlay very hilly terrain. Even though most of the sites here attract tent campers, as they are smaller and on steep hills, a few RVs park here on the 13 electric sites. Many of the sites overlook a different cove of Kentucky Lake than Area A. Some sites have been leveled, some not. A bathhouse stands on this hilltop, along a spur road with campsites that do not have a lake view. A dock and boat ramp make fishing convenient for anglers. A fish-cleaning station also attracts anglers to this area. Note that the loop with sites 36–47 is a 24-hour generator operation area.

Area T, with 50 campsites, is landlocked. It fills first since it has electricity, water, and sewer hookups. Senior campers prefer this tight-knit series of concentric loops beneath the pines with a grassy understory. A shower and bathroom is in the center of the loops.

Area D, with 62 electric and water sites, fills up fast. The sites are heavily shaded but are also small and cramped. There is nothing but pavement and gravel beneath the trees. Get friendly with your neighbors here, as you will be seeing a lot of them.

Area C, with 115 sites, is newer and more appealing. The campsites offer more spaciousness beneath widespread oaks and cedars. Most sites offer water and electricity; 17 sites have water, electricity, and sewer. The many lakeside sites go first. The sites farthest from the lake are basic. Some overlook Dodds Creek, which flows into Kentucky Lake. Others are on a hillside and are used by tent campers. A newer bathhouse centers the loop. Showers are available to noncampers for a small fee.

The campground attracts active family campers, young folks riding mountain bikes, anglers, and retirees. Hillman Ferry can fill up quickly, especially on summer holiday weekends. Nice summer weekends will fill the sites, but summer weekdays will see sites available. The more developed the site, the sooner it will fill. Hillman Ferry mostly attracts RVs, though tents and pop-ups are well represented.

Activities are nearly limitless. In summer, the Forest Service has on-site naturalists offering outdoor programs to keep kids busy. A campground swim beach offers watery fun for the younger set. Adults make their own fun. Many will be using the two campground ramps to launch their boats in search of fish on Kentucky Lake. Others will be water skiing or gunning personal watercraft.

A softball field, archery range, and game court offer outdoor recreation on land. Still others will be enjoying some of the area trails. The Hillman Heritage National Recreation Trail is a 5.5-mile series of interconnected loops that follows historic roads of the Star Lime Works community. Interpretive information along the trails enhances the experience. Other interconnected paved trails leave the campground from Area T. The North Paved Trail leaves from the campground entrance road and heads 1.5 miles to the North Welcome Station. The North–South Trail is also open to hikers and mountain bikers, offering loop possibilities. The Canal Loop Trail offers 14 more miles of pathways for hikers and bikers.

Pets are allowed but must be leashed, and all of their waste should be cleaned up. The Hillman Ferry Outpost rents mountain and cruiser bikes and camping equipment. They also have a limited food selection oriented toward campers, like hot dog buns, coffee, and convenience items. Soft-drink machines are also at the campground. Ice, firewood, and tick repellent can be purchased at the gatehouse. To contact the gatehouse for other information, call 270-924-2181. A limited number of campsites are available for seasonal camping, ranging from two to nine months. Call well ahead for details.

ACCESS From the North Welcome Station, head south on Woodlands Trace 1.5 miles to Forest Road 110. Turn right on FR 110 and follow it to dead-end at the campground entrance station.

■ PINEY

NEAREST TOWN Dover, TN   **OPEN** March–November   **INDIVIDUAL SITES** 316 sites with electrical hookups; 44 sites with electric, water, and sewer; 24 primitive sites; 9 small cabins   **EACH SITE** Picnic table, fire grate; some have lantern posts; others varying combination of electric, water, and sewer   **SITE ASSIGNMENT** First come, first served and by reservation; 800-525-7077, or online at **landbetweenthelakes.us/reservations**   **REGISTRATION** At campground gatehouse   **FACILITIES** Hot showers, water spigots, camp store   **FEE** Yes, rates rise with varying combinations of electric, water, and sewer at site

THREE HUNDRED EIGHTY-FOUR can be a scary number. At least when you are talking about the number of campsites in a campground. This usually spells an overcrowded city of tents, pop-ups, and RVs in a world of congestion, mayhem, and all the things from which you are trying to get away. Piney, however, bucks the trend. This getaway on the southwest side of LBL has numerous loops spread over a wide acreage. A competent staff keeps things organized, so you can concentrate on having a good time. Recreational opportunities are many and varied: boating, hiking, fishing, and historical study.

Pass the entrance kiosk and enter the campground. Eight loops comprise Piney Campground. Black Oak Loop is situated on a peninsula jutting into Kentucky Lake and has 92 campsites spread out along three loops. Thirty or so sites enjoy lake frontage, where campers pull up their boats. Some of this frontage is on a small lake cove, as opposed to the main lake. Hickory-oak woodland shades the widely separated sites. The large campsites have been leveled, but scant understory undermines campsite privacy. Small, wet-weather drainages break up the terrain. A grassy area lies between the campground and a swim beach. One of the two bathhouses has showers.

The Chestnut Loop also has many lakefront and waterfront sites that overlook the swim beach. The sites are very spacious. Four camping shelters grace this loop. The Dogwood Loop, with full hookups, is always busy with RVs. The other loops will be generally half RV, half tent, even on the electric loops. The sites in Persimmon Loop are a little close together but do have the coveted lakefront sites. Many of the other sites are open to the sun.

The Sweetgum Loop has 34 sites. Most sites at the beginning are inside the loop. Swing by the lake and come to some fine sites overlooking the water, about 30 feet from the water. The end of the loop has some decent sites that are a little crowded. The Virginia Loop does not have electricity and thus is the realm of the tent campers. With 24 sites shaded by pines and oaks, the loop descends toward the water. Six waterside sites here are some of the best in the entire campground. Other sites here are a little too cramped for my taste. The end of the loop has ultrashady sites. Water spigots are strategically situated throughout both loops. A fully equipped bathhouse serves both loops. Showers are available to noncampers for a small fee.

The campground has family campers on weekends and seniors during the week. Most everyone who comes here, especially in the summer, is water oriented. Active campers are scattered throughout the week. Piney generally fills on summer holiday weekends. Other times, you should have no trouble getting a site. Waterfront sites go first, especially for campers with boats. The full hookup sites go next. The nonelectric basic sites are the last to fill. Piney has long-term campsites available for seasonal rentals.

Small cabins can also be rented. These shelters sleep four and include a double bed, bunk bed, ceiling fan, and electrical outlets. Shelter renters use the campground bathhouses for restrooms and showers. They are reservable the same way as are campsites. An on-site store, the Outpost, has camping supplies and food. The Outpost also rents camping supplies ranging from tents and lanterns to coolers and fishing poles. You could actually come to Piney empty-handed and go on a camping trip! This is good for campers who are short on gear. Call the campground at 931-232-5331 for rental rates and long-term camping information.

Now, what to do? Go boating on Kentucky Lake, fish at the all-access pier, fish without a boat at Catfish Pond, or dip yourself in the water at the swim beach.

Piney has 2 miles of trail reserved for the sole use of its campers. This trail network begins at the campground gatehouse. The paved portion of the trail makes a 1.3-mile loop. An additional 0.7-mile subloop is made of gravel and dirt. It curves along a peninsula of the lake and is open to hikers and bikers.

The campground roads are great for biking. Bikes are available for rent at the camp store. Better yet, bring your own two-wheeler. Hikers have the Fort Henry Trails to tackle. There are 29 miles of paths here and you can actually trace Ulysses S. Grant's movements between Fort Henry and nearby Fort Donelson. These forts were the sites of the first Civil War attacks on the river routes in the war's western theater. A Fort Henry Trail map reveals numerous loop possibilities. The Piney Trail leads from near the campground into this trail network.

Fort Donelson, just a few miles away on the Cumberland River, is a national battlefield where the star of Ulysses S. Grant first rose. You can tour the battlefield by walking 7.0 miles of interpretive trails or by travel by auto. Check out the river battery, where big guns are located, and the still-standing Dover Hotel, where the losing side surrendered.

ACCESS   From the South Welcome Station, take Fort Henry Road, Forest Road 230, for 8.0 miles to the Piney Campground entrance road. Turn right on the entrance road and enter the campground.

SPECIAL-USE CAMPGROUNDS
For Campers with Specific Interests

■ TURKEY BAY OHV AREA

NEAREST TOWN Aurora, KY   **OPEN** Year-round   **INDIVIDUAL SITES** Unspecified   **EACH SITE** Sites are basic, some have picnic tables   **SITE ASSIGNMENT** First come, first served   **REGISTRATION** On site   **FACILITIES** Water, vault toilets   **FEE** Yes, camping fee is in addition to off-highway vehicle (OHV) user permit.

TURKEY BAY OFF-HIGHWAY VEHICLE AREA was the first federal off-high-way camping and riding area in the nation. This is just one more unique aspect of LBL. In this 2,500-acre swath of land near Kentucky Lake, OHV riders can drive their vehicles along the ridges and valleys to their hearts' content. This concept, in keeping with LBL's multiple-use ideology, concentrates usage in one area. And when OHVers aren't riding, they can camp with their fellow riders, swapping trail tales.

Leave Woodlands Trace and enter Turkey Bay OHV. Immediately reach the registration booth. You can register your OHV here (a must), or at Golden Pond Visitor Center if the booth isn't open. A water spigot is nearby. Many day users park near here, unload their four wheelers (four-wheel-drive autos are allowed as well), and take off. A few campsites with picnic tables are set beside a line of trees, but the area can be muddy or dusty. Continue on Forest Road 167, which is the southern OHV-area boundary, and shortly reach the primary camping and unloading area. This area is rockier. Campsites, some shaded, some not, are irregularly dispersed on both sides of the road. Some of the campsites have picnic tables. Off-highway vehicle trails spur off the road to the north near the portable toilets and unloading ramps.

FR 167 reaches a field. Campsites are on the edge of the woods beside the field. Pass a hill then reach another flat that overlooks the lake. This is the 24-hour generator area, meaning all who camp back here can run their generators anytime, day or night.

Folks come from everywhere to enjoy this resource. It sees use year-round, but is busier in the warm season. OHV riders exclusively use the Turkey Bay Campground, though anyone can camp back here. If you aren't an OHV enthusiast, you are better off camping elsewhere.

The Turkey Creek watershed was chosen as the OHV area due to its being rockier than most valleys, allowing for less erosion and siltation of the streams. Riders have established trails and a permit is required to use them. You can purchase either an annual permit or a three-day permit. Finally, a liability waiver form must be filled out and is available at **landbetweenthelakes.us.** See the website for a map of the area and the latest riding rules, which are strictly enforced.

ACCESS   From the entrance of Golden Pond Visitor Center, take Woodlands Trace south 1.8 miles to FR 167. Turn right on FR 167 and enter the OHV area.

■ WRANGLERS CAMPGROUND

NEAREST TOWN Canton, KY   **OPEN** Year-round   **INDIVIDUAL SITES** 203, 12 cabins   **EACH SITE** Picnic table, fire grate, some have varying combinations of electric, water, and sewer   **SITE ASSIGNMENT** First come, first served and by reservation; 800-525-7077, or online at **landbetweenthelakes.us/reservations**   **REGISTRATION** At gatehouse   **FACILITIES** Hot showers, flush toilets, water spigots, laundry, camp store, restaurant, riding stables. For horses: hay, stables, picket poles and/or hitches, watering troughs, washing stations, farrier/blacksmith   **FEE** Yes, rates rise with varying combinations of electric, water, and sewer at site   **OTHER** Bicycles expressly forbidden in the campground

WRANGLERS CAMPGROUND IS a good idea that has been well implemented. This campground is designed for, but not exclusive to, horseback riders. The whole area is geared around the equestrian set. The campground is large, not only because it has more than 200 sites, but also because of the riding stables, horse barns and stables, restaurant, and camping shelters, known here as bunkhouses. Situated in the wide valley of lower Lick Creek, the area is a village unto its own. And the horseback riders have a set of trails unto their own, a set that includes 100 miles of marked paths. The trails start at Wranglers Campground, thus equestrians can combine camping with riding in the hub of equestrian life at LBL.

Enter the LBL's only horse-camp campground at the gatehouse. This wooden structure is full of friendly people aiming to help. If you have never been here before, they will look at your rig, ask your camping preferences, and send you to a site you will probably like. If you have been here before, they'll try to put you on the site you

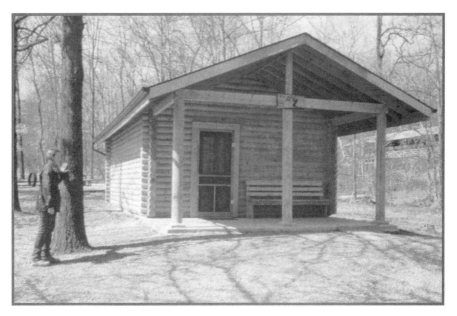

Camping shelter at Wranglers Campground

choose. The campsites can be reserved, so if you find one suitable for your desires, note it then reserve it the next go-round.

The campground is open year-round. In winter, use is weather dependent. Wranglers is the only full-facility campground open in the cold months, and non-equestrians sometimes end up here. Occasionally, users of the Turkey Bay OHV Area will camp here to enjoy the full facilities. Occupancy picks up when spring warms, peaking around Memorial Day. Early summer is busy, but use dips in the dog days of summer. When September hits, the campground fills again and stays busy until the leaves fall and frost covers the ground. Hunters camp here in winter. Campers will be seen in tents, pop-ups, and RVs. But most Wranglers Camp users will be in something unique to the equestrian set—combination horse trailers with living quarters. Generally, campers prefer sites that are convenient to both a bathhouse and a barn.

Enter the campground and pass the day-use area on the right. Riding stables are located here for those without horses who want guided rides. Equestrians who come for the day park their rigs here. Ahead are three of the cabins. More cabins are scattered throughout the campground. They stay busy, and reservations are recommended. The bunkhouses have a bed, ceiling fan and light, table and benches, and electrical outlet inside. Small heaters are available for winter. Outside are the porch, a fire ring, and a picnic table. Shelter campers use the bathhouses. Speaking of bathhouses, showers are available to noncampers for a small fee. Bathhouses and water spigots are evenly spread around Wranglers Camp, as are stalls and watering troughs for horses. Most campsites have a tethering post if you choose to keep your horse at your campsite. Seven barns with 160 stalls are available for a fee. Bring your own hose if you want to use the concrete horse-washing areas. Disconnect your hose after you are done.

Enter Area A. The first sites here, up on a hill, offer seasonal camping. Call the campground office for details. All sites in A have electricity. Some have water, electric, and sewer hookups. The Outpost is in the center of A. It offers food, supplies, and horse tack. They also have a restaurant inside. A picnic shelter and playground are also within this fenced spot. Area B is farther up the hollow and has a mix of sun and shade, all with electricity. These sites are popular. Even farther up the hollow is Area G. These basic sites have only a picnic table and fire ring. The lack of pads keeps trailers away. Campers with smaller setups seek this area, which offers the most solitude.

Area C is at the lower end of Lick Hollow. This was originally a hay field, but is now planted with trees. Shade is limited among these 58 sites. You can look out from here and see the hills encircling the Lick Creek Valley. Area C is the first camping area visible from the entrance.

Pass the farrier/blacksmith barn. The operator is on site most weekends. Come to Area D, known as "The Pines." Pine trees have been planted in the center of the loop and provide shade. This area is coveted in summer. All 46 sites have electricity. A side road leaves to the overflow camp area. It is just a big field, but equestrian campers should know that no one is ever turned away, even if all official sites are taken.

Area E is stretched along a line of trees and has a miniloop at the end. Groups gather in the miniloop for activities. Area F is set between Area D and Area A. It offers 15 basic sites open to the sun. A large, grassy hill centers the loop.

Once camp is set up, horse lovers like to ride the trails. Others will bring wagons to ride the trails. Some just like to amble around the camp. Equestrian trails have been laid out, exploring the oak ridges, hardwood bottoms, and all points in between. All four trailheads leave from Wranglers Camp, and all trails are named and numbered. Loops range from 3 to 14 miles in length. The trails are interconnected, making loop combinations unlimited. Picnic tables, hitching facilities, and trash receptacles are situated at popular resting spots along the trails. A trail map is available online and at the gatehouse.

LBL staff offer interpretive programs on some weekends. Special events are held at Wranglers annually. In July, the LBL Primitive Rodeo extends over two evenings and is very popular. The Grand Jubilee, a tribute to campers, is also in July. In September, the American Trail Riders Association event draws folks from all over the country. If you are an equestrian, you couldn't ask for much more than is offered here at Wranglers.

ACCESS From the entrance of Golden Pond Visitor Center, take Woodlands Trace south 0.2 mile to paved Forest Road 165. Turn left on FR 165 and follow it 5.0 miles to an intersection. FR 166 keeps forward. Turn right here, as FR 165 shortly reaches Wranglers Campground.

For Groups

■ BRANDON SPRINGS GROUP CENTER

NEAREST TOWN Dover, TN   **OPEN** Year-round   **REGISTRATION** Must be reserved in advance; call 270-924-2044   **FACILITIES** Dorms, commons building with kitchen staff, activity building, amphitheater, swimming beach, hiking trails, campfire areas   **FEE** Call, depends on number of dorms being used, will accommodate up to 128 people

BRANDON SPRINGS IS a high-quality, well-kept facility. It was built for groups interested in the environmental educational opportunities at LBL. It is used for educational as well as social events by school groups, church groups, scouts, and for family reunions.

Situated on the shores of Bards Lake, the buildings are stretched along the shoreline, offering an appealing atmosphere. Numerous activities and facilities are on site. Users at Brandon Springs can canoe Bards Lake, hike a trail system exclusive for their use, or use the fishing pier. They can enjoy the swimming pool or swim beach on Bards Lake. Hard-surfaced courts are available for games, and a mown recreation field is on site for lawn games. LBL interpretive rangers offer numerous outdoor education programs, ranging from outdoor survival skills to orienteering to nature study. These nature study programs cover the animals, streams, ponds, insects, and nightlife of LBL.

To reserve Brandon Springs, start with a call to the number above. They have a specific yet not-too-complicated reservation system. The facility can be reserved up to a year in advance. Spring and fall are the most popular times, due to school group use. Winter is the least used time.

ACCESS From the South Welcome Station, take Woodlands Trace north 2.2 miles and turn right on paved Forest Road 226. Follow FR 226 to dead-end at the facility.

■ COLSON HOLLOW GROUP CAMPGROUND

NEAREST TOWN Aurora, KY **OPEN** Year-round **INDIVIDUAL SITES** Unspecified **EACH SITE** Access to picnic tables and grills shared by group members **SITE ASSIGNMENT** By reservation **REGISTRATION** Must be reserved in advance; call 270-924-2044 **FACILITIES** Picnic tables, electricity, accessible vault toilets **FEE** Call, depends on group size

COLSON HOLLOW GROUP Camp lies in an isolated bay on the shores of Kentucky Lake. It was put here to allow large groups plenty of solitude to endeavor in their desired pursuits. Everybody from motorcycle groups to scouts to church organizations stay here. The large area will accommodate groups of up to 200.

Gravel Forest Road 169 crosses the streambed that forms the hollow and enters a field big enough to swallow two or three football fields. Kentucky Lake is open to the west. Immediately to your left is a group of picnic tables shaded by a scattering of large hardwoods. The campground road bisects the field and reaches a line of trees on the far side. More picnic tables lie on the edge of the woods. The campground road continues toward the lake and slips around to a smaller hollow broken with trees. An electricity outlet is located here and is available to campers who have bands or speakers. This is the most popular camping area. Portable toilets are also located here.

Groups using the camp most often conduct their own activities. Nearby activities offered in the LBL include hiking the North–South Trail, fishing Kentucky Lake, visiting The Homeplace and the Bison Range, and visiting the Golden Pond Visitor Center with its planetarium show.

ACCESS From the entrance to Golden Pond Visitor Center, take Woodlands Trace south 3.1 miles and turn right on FR 169. Follow FR 169 2.0 miles to dead-end at the campground.

Nearby State Parks
KENLAKE STATE RESORT PARK

KENTUCKY'S KENLAKE STATE Resort Park is highly developed, much like Tennessee's Paris Landing. Back in the 1940s, the Tennessee Valley Authority bought land near Eggners Ferry Bridge then deeded it over to Kentucky. The commonwealth made it a state park. Facilities were built, including a hotel, and Kentucky had its first resort state park.

Located a few miles west of the heart of LBL, the state has packed the park with a variety of things, including a dining room, golf course, cottages, marina, picnic shelter, playground, campground, and some trails. The most unusual facility is an indoor tennis center. Outdoor courts are also available for warm-weather play.

The campground is a 90-site affair open April–October. All the sites have water and electrical hookups. A fully equipped bathhouse and a dump station make life easy on campers. However, there is a problem. The campground is bordered on two sides by roads and only one side by the lake. However, the lakeside sites do offer bluff-top views of Kentucky Lake. Come here if you want the more modernized version of "roughing it."

ACCESS   From the entrance to the Golden Pond Visitor Center, drive south a quarter mile to Golden Pond Road. Turn left on Golden Pond Road and follow it 0.3 mile to US 68/KY 80. Turn left, heading west, and follow US 68/KY 80 4.2 miles, crossing over Kentucky Lake to the state park. The campground is on your right and the balance of the park is to your left.

KENTUCKY DAM VILLAGE STATE RESORT PARK

THIS PARK BOASTS of having the most choices for overnight accommodations in the state park system, with the largest marina on the largest lake in the state of Kentucky. Located on the west side of Kentucky Lake near Kentucky Dam, the park has a lodge, an inn, and 72 cottages. The campground has 221 sites, in addition to the air campground, where you can camp by your plane! All of this is true. If you are looking to live high while visiting Land Between The Lakes, this state park may be your choice.

Many roads cut through the Kentucky Dam Village, which cuts into the rustic atmosphere. But the lodge and cottages are quality. The large dining room offers breakfast, lunch, and dinner. Enjoy these accommodations. They are your best bet for incorporating this park into your LBL visit. However, if you are looking to camp, skip this campground. It is below the par set by the rest of the park. The large campground is in a mostly open flat set apart from the lake and the rest of the state park. Campgrounds inside LBL offer a better setting. Kentucky Dam Village does have a golf course, and its marina is open March–October. You can dock your boat overnight or rent watercraft from pontoon boats to wave runners. The marina is a good piece from the campground.

A swim beach on Kentucky Lake appeals to sunbathers and children. Playgrounds and picnic areas overlook the lake. Tennis and shuffleboard courts round out the outdoor recreation. On-site naturalists offer programs for children and adults.

ACCESS   Kentucky Dam Village State Resort Park is located northwest of Grand Rivers, KY, on the west side of Kentucky Dam where US 62 and US 621 split.

LAKE BARKLEY STATE RESORT PARK

THIS STATE PARK, a few miles east of the heart of LBL, has some pretty acreage. Set on the Little River Arm of Lake Barkley, its facilities are situated in a mix of high ridges, steep hollows, and lakeside flats. And it has many facilities: two lodges, cottages, fitness center, golf course, even its own airport! To its credit, most of the facilities are tastefully integrated into the attractive landscape. The lake is the star of the show. To better enjoy the lake, the park offers a marina, large boat ramp, and swim beach.

The campground is set on a bluff above Lake Barkley. It is open year-round. All 79 sites have a picnic table, grill, and electricity. Hot showers, flush toilets, and a laundry facility are on site. The heavily shaded campground has a mossy understory. Some sites overlook the lake. The far side of the loop has more widely spaced sites but no lake view. The campground has its own boat ramp, albeit steep.

The park has a trail system to explore the nature preserve in the park's interior. However, the park is more oriented toward developed recreation. If you are looking for a developed resort state park, this is the best of the bunch around LBL.

ACCESS From the entrance to the Golden Pond Visitor Center, drive south a quarter mile to Golden Pond Road. Turn left on Golden Pond Road and follow it 0.3 miles to US 68/KY 80. Turn right, heading east, and follow US 68/KY 80 7.8 miles, crossing over Lake Barkley along the way to reach KY 1489. Turn left on KY 1489 and follow it 2.0 miles to the park. Keep forward past the right turn to the golf course to reach the balance of the facilities.

PARIS LANDING STATE RESORT PARK

PARIS LANDING STATE Resort Park is one of Tennessee's seven premier resort parks. Situated on the western side of Kentucky Lake near the southwestern end of LBL, this highly developed getaway tries to offer something for everybody. It has an inn overlooking Kentucky Lake, a conference center, marina, cabins, campground, ball fields, golf course, picnic areas galore, swimming pool, and restaurant.

The lake is the big draw. Water skiers, anglers, and sailboaters use the marina. Anglers can fish by boat or from the park pier. The campground is stuck between the marina and US 79, making it less than rustic. A couple of hiking trails course through the park, but hikers are better off using the LBL trails. You can enjoy Paris Landing if you have a big boat and want to use the marina, or if you want to stay at the inn and eat a big meal at their restaurant.

ACCESS Paris Landing State Resort Park is 11 miles west of Dover, TN, on US 79 South just over the Kentucky Lake bridge.

▪ Appendixes ▪

Resources

FRIENDS OF LAND BETWEEN THE LAKES

345 Maintenance Road
Golden Pond, KY 42211
800-455-5897, 270-924-2007
friendsoflbl.org

THIS PHILANTHROPIC GROUP formed in 1983 and originally partnered with the Tennessee Valley Authority when it ran Land Between The Lakes. However, since the U.S. Forest Service took over management of LBL in 1999, the role of Friends of LBL has expanded and they "provide program services, fund development, and help promote the wise and sustainable use of the Land Between The Lakes." Their efforts extend from providing funding for specific projects to ongoing management of facilities. They are a force for good at LBL and welcome new members and business partners. Please visit their website to join the Friends of LBL or learn more about their operations.

OTHER RESOURCES

Volunteering

LAND BETWEEN THE LAKES NATIONAL RECREATION AREA needs your help! The United States Forest Service, which manages the recreation area, can always use some extra help. Volunteering is a rewarding way to give back to the places that you love. Not only are individuals encouraged to get involved, but so are groups. According to the Friends of LBL website, "volunteer activities range from trail maintenance and cleanup, to support of special events, monitoring the Elk & Bison Prairie, or assisting with administrative work. Volunteering is a great way to have a meaningful and rewarding experience in the great outdoors at Land Between The Lakes." Volunteer work positions are available. Contact Friends of Land Between The Lakes at **friendsoflbl.org** or 270-924-2007.

Contact List

LAND BETWEEN THE LAKES NATIONAL RECREATION AREA
100 Van Morgan Drive
Golden Pond, KY 42211
800-lbl-7077
landbetweenthelakes.us

FORT DONELSON NATIONAL BATTLEFIELD
P.O. Box 434
Dover, TN 24354
931-232-5706
nps.gov/fodo

KENLAKE STATE RESORT PARK
542 Kenlake Road
Hardin, KY 42048
270-474-2211
parks.ky.gov

KENTUCKY DAM VILLAGE STATE RESORT PARK
113 Administration Drive
Gilbertsville, KY 42044
270-362-4271
parks.ky.gov

LAKE BARKLEY STATE RESORT PARK
3500 State Park Road
Cadiz, KY 42211
270-924-1131
parks.ky.gov

PARIS LANDING STATE RESORT PARK
Route 1
Buchanan, TN 38222
901-644-7359
tnstateparks.com

Index

About the Author

JOHNNY MOLLOY IS a writer and adventurer based in Tennessee. His outdoor passion ignited on a backpacking trip in Great Smoky Mountains National Park while attending the University of Tennessee. That first foray unleashed a love of the outdoors that led Johnny to spend over 3,500 nights backpacking, canoe camping, and tent camping throughout the country over the past three decades.

Friends enjoyed his outdoor adventure stories; one even suggested he write a book. He pursued his friend's idea and soon parlayed his love of the outdoors into an

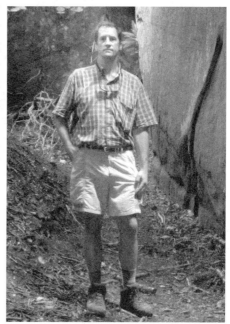

occupation. The results of his efforts are more than 50 books and guides. His writings include hiking guidebooks, camping guidebooks, paddling guidebooks, comprehensive guidebooks about a specific area, and true outdoor adventure books all over the eastern United States.

Though primarily involved with book publications, Molloy writes for various magazines, for websites, and is an outdoors columnist and feature writer for his local paper, the *Johnson City Press*. He continues writing and traveling extensively throughout the United States, endeavoring in a variety of outdoor pursuits. For the latest on Johnny, please visit **johnnymolloy.com.**

Check out this great title from
— Menasha Ridge Press! —

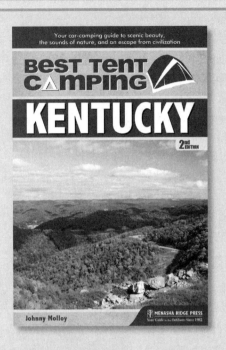

Your car-camping guide to scenic beauty, the sounds of nature, and an escape from civilization

BEST TENT CAMPING
KENTUCKY
2nd EDITION

Johnny Molloy

MENASHA RIDGE PRESS
Your Guide to the Outdoors Since 1982

Best Tent Camping:
Kentucky

by Johnny Molloy

ISBN: 978-1-63404-004-4

$15.95, 2nd Edition

6x9, paperback

192 pages

B&W photos, maps

This guide, by author Johnny Molloy, leads you to the best tent camping destinations within these parcels of the Bluegrass State, describing not only the campgrounds themselves but also the fun outdoorsy activities nearby. The guide uses a rating system that measures campground privacy, security, beauty, quiet, and cleanliness, and gives inside tips on how to enjoy each particular destination from your chosen campground. It also details prices, opening and closing dates, websites, and other information that will help you make the most of your Kentucky tent camping experience.

MENASHA RIDGE PRESS
www.menasharidge.com
Your Guide to the Outdoors Since 1982